T0183472

Lecture Notes in Computer Science   10126

Commenced Publication in 1973
Founding and Former Series Editors:
Gerhard Goos, Juris Hartmanis, and Jan van Leeuwen

More information about this series at http://www.springer.com/series/7412

Martin Reuter · Christian Wachinger
Hervé Lombaert (Eds.)

Spectral and Shape Analysis in Medical Imaging

First International Workshop, SeSAMI 2016
Held in Conjunction with MICCAI 2016
Athens, Greece, October 21, 2016
Revised Selected Papers

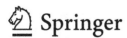 Springer

Editors
Martin Reuter
Harvard Medical School
Boston, MA
USA

Hervé Lombaert
Inria Sophia Antipolis
Sophia Antipolis
France

Christian Wachinger
Ludwig-Maximilian University of Munich
Munich
Germany

ISSN 0302-9743 ISSN 1611-3349 (electronic)
Lecture Notes in Computer Science
ISBN 978-3-319-51236-5 ISBN 978-3-319-51237-2 (eBook)
DOI 10.1007/978-3-319-51237-2

Library of Congress Control Number: 2016960313

LNCS Sublibrary: SL6 – Image Processing, Computer Vision, Pattern Recognition, and Graphics

Printed on acid-free paper

This Springer imprint is published by Springer Nature
The registered company is Springer International Publishing AG
The registered company address is: Gewerbestrasse 11, 6330 Cham, Switzerland

Preface

This volume contains the proceedings of the First International Workshop on Spectral and Shape Analysis in Medical Imaging (SeSAMI 2016) held on October 21, 2016, in Athens, Greece, in conjunction with the 19th International Conference on Medical Image Computing and Computer Assisted Interventions (MICCAI 2016). This workshop is an extension of the Spectral Analysis in Medical Imaging (SAMI) workshop held at MICCAI 2015.

Today's image data often represent continuous and time-varying phenomena, usually with a geometric structure. Shape and geometry processing methods are, therefore, starting to receive increased attention, for example, due to their higher sensitivity to local variations relative to traditional markers, such as the volume of a structure. In medical image computing or computer-aided interventions in particular, the understanding of shapes and their geometrical representations enables the modeling of organs from an anatomical as well as a functional perspective.

Moreover, spectral methods provide a wealth of opportunities for studying complex data. They support the analyses by helping to understand high-dimensional structures representing population or disease data and are often combined with shape analysis due to their properties, such as isometry invariance. Both shape and spectral analysis have, therefore, found many applications in medical image analysis.

This workshop provided an invaluable opportunity for researchers to present recent work on spectral and shape analysis, as well as methods at the intersection of these domains, and consisted of two components. The first focused on theoretical aspects and state-of-the-art research on spectral analysis and the characterization of shape in the form of talks and invited expert presentations. The second focused on cutting-edge research on medical image applications in the form of oral presentations of accepted submissions. Novel and original submissions were encouraged on emerging approaches with topics including segmentation, registration, and classification.

We are extremely grateful to the contributors of this SeSAMI workshop. We thank all authors who shared their latest findings, as well as the Program Committee members, and reviewers, who all achieved quality work in a very short time. We also thank our keynote speakers, who kindly accepted our invitations: Guido Gerig, Professor at the New York University, USA, and Tom Fletcher, Professor at the University of Utah, USA.

November 2016

Hervé Lombaert
Christian Wachinger
Martin Reuter

Organization

Organizing Committee

Martin Reuter   Harvard Medical School, Boston, MA, USA
Christian Wachinger   Ludwig Maximilian University, Munich, Germany
Hervé Lombaert   Inria, France and University of Quebec (ETS), Canada

Program Committee

Stanley Durrleman   Inria, France
Guido Gerig   New York University, USA
Ender Konukoglu   ETH Zurich, Switzerland
Julien Lefevre   Université Aix-Marseille, France
Diana Mateus   Technische Universität München, Germany
Washington Mio   Florida State University, USA
Marc Niethammer   UNC Chapel Hill, USA
Stephen Pizer   UNC Chapel Hill, USA
Robert Pless   Washington University, USA
Kilian Pohl   SRI, USA
Yonggang Shi   University of Southern California, USA
Martin Styner   UNC Chapel Hill, USA
Ross Whitaker   University of Utah, USA

Sponsoring Institutions

Inria Sophia-Antipolis, France
Ludwig Maximilian University, Munich, Germany
Harvard Medical School, Boston, MA, USA

Contents

Spectral Methods

A Volumetric Conformal Mapping Approach for Clustering White Matter Fibers in the Brain

Vikash Gupta[1]([⊠]), Gautam Prasad[2], and Paul Thompson[1]

[1] Imaging Genetics Center, University of Southern California, Los Angeles, USA
contact@vikashgupta.net
[2] Google Inc., Los Angeles, USA

Abstract. The human brain may be considered as a genus-0 shape, topologically equivalent to a sphere. Various methods have been used in the past to transform the brain surface to that of a sphere using harmonic energy minimization methods used for cortical surface matching. However, very few methods have studied volumetric parameterization of the brain using a spherical embedding. Volumetric parameterization is typically used for complicated geometric problems like shape matching, morphing and isogeometric analysis. Using conformal mapping techniques, we can establish a bijective mapping between the brain and the topologically equivalent sphere. Our hypothesis is that shape analysis problems are simplified when the shape is defined in an intrinsic coordinate system. Our goal is to establish such a coordinate system for the brain. The efficacy of the method is demonstrated with a white matter clustering problem. Initial results show promise for future investigation in these parameterization technique and its application to other problems related to computational anatomy like registration and segmentation.

Keywords: Conformal mapping · Volumetric parameterization · Spectral clustering · White matter fiber clustering

1 Introduction

Shape parameterization is a well researched area in the computational geometry community [1,2]. In computational anatomy, many algorithms have been devoted to surface parameterization [3–6] and its applications to cortical surface matching and registration [7]. Shi et al. [8] used conformal mapping between the cortical surfaces for cortical label fusion. Brain Transfer [9] is a recent method suggested by Lombaert et al. is used to find correspondences between cortical surface across subjects as well as functional areas. Surface parameterization may be sufficient for analyzing surface geometry. However, it falls short when there is significant information contained inside the shape under consideration (brain). Here we developed a parameterization technique that parameterizes the entire volume of the brain and every structure contained in it. Thus, cortical surface parameterization is in fact a byproduct of this method.

© Springer International Publishing AG 2016
M. Reuter et al. (Eds.): SeSAMI 2016, LNCS 10126, pp. 3–14, 2016.
DOI: 10.1007/978-3-319-51237-2_1

Following work by Wang and colleagues [10] using "sphere carving" to harmonically map the brain to a sphere, a bijective mapping between the brain and the topologically equivalent sphere can be established using a 3D harmonic function. Such a parameterization gives us a coordinate system intrinsic to the brain shape, which may simplify various sub-problems related to computational anatomy such as registration, segmentation and automated clustering of white matter fibers. We will show a potential application of this parameterization technique, to assist with automated clustering of white matter fibers.

White matter fibers serve as neural pathways that connect different parts of the brain. Diffusion weighted imaging (DWI) and tractography are used to study the white matter organization in the brain. Clustering the white matter fibers is an important step towards statistical analyses. One commonly used clustering method [11] uses manual ROI delineation on the FA images. These regions can be used to seed whole-brain fiber tractography, which is then grouped into white matter bundles using spectral clustering. One method used Hausdorff's distance [12] as a distance metric between two fibers. Another more recent method for fiber clustering was proposed by [13]. In this method, each fiber is represented using Gaussian mixture models followed by a hierarchical total Bregman soft clustering. The authors [14] provide a more complete overview of different clustering techniques.

In this paper, we use the proposed conformal mapping technique to parameterize the white matter tracks. We then use a hierarchical spectral clustering approach to classify a given set of tracks into individual anatomically relevant fiber bundles. The proposed method does not rely on any tractography atlas or region of interest (ROI) information. The accuracy of the method is compared with manual clustering results.

2   Conformal Mapping: A Heat Transfer Analogy

To understand the volumetric parameterization problem addressed in this paper, we draw an analogy between our problem and the heat transfer problem in solid bodies. For the purpose of explanation, consider a solid body is maintained at a constant high temperature on the surface and at another point inside the brain at a constant low temperature. At steady state a thermal gradient will be set up between the surface and the center with different layers of isothermal surfaces. The heat from the high temperature surface is conducted towards the center through heat-flow lines. These heat-flow lines intersect the isothermal surfaces at right angles. We use this property to define a coordinate system for the whole brain. We refer to the fixed low temperature point as the *shapecenter* and the temperature field as ϕ.

3   Harmonic Function

The harmonic function is a C^2 continuous function that satisfies Laplace's equation. It is used to establish a bijective mapping between the brain and the topologically equivalent spherical shape. If $\phi : U \rightarrow R^n$, where $U \subseteq R^n$ is some domain and ϕ is some function defined over U, the function ϕ is harmonic if its Laplacian vanishes over U, i.e., $\nabla^2 \phi = 0$. In terms of Cartesian coordinate system, we can write

$$\nabla^2 \phi = \sum_{i=1}^{n} \frac{\partial^2 \phi}{\partial^2 x_i} = 0 \tag{1}$$

where x_i is the ith Cartesian coordinate and n is the number of dimensions of the shape under study (here, 3). The harmonic function has two properties called the mean value and the maximum principle property, which are important for the parameterization problem being discussed.

3.1   Mean Value Property

If a ball $B(x, r)$ with center x and radius r is completely contained within the domain under study, then the value of the harmonic function $\phi(x)$ is given by the average values of the function over the surface of the sphere. This average value is also equal to the average values of ϕ inside the sphere.

3.2   Maximum Principle

According to the maximum principle, the harmonic function ϕ cannot have local extrema within the domain U. The Laplacian of the harmonic functions should be zero by definition. For a local extremum to exist all the components of the second order partial derivatives of the function should have the same sign. If all of them have the same sign, their sum will never be zero and thus they will never be able to satisfy Laplace's equation.

4   Algorithm

For the parameterization method, the volume generated by the fractional anisotropy (FA) mask is used. Image voxels were classified as either boundary surface points or internal points. For every subject the inferior end of the fornix on the midline was located manually and designated as the "shape center". In the future, more automated approach towards choosing the same will be investigated and adopted.

4.1   Boundary Conditions

We apply the Dirchlet boundary conditions for the shapecenter and the boundary surface, i.e., we fix the value of the function ϕ on all the boundary nodes and the shapecenter to 1 and 0 respectively. All the remaining points are assigned random values between 0 and 1 as the initial condition.

4.2 Potential Computation

An iterative finite difference scheme is used to solve the Laplace equations. If $\phi(x, y, z)$ is a harmonic function, its second derivative is computed using the Taylor's series expansion.

$$\frac{\partial^2 \phi}{\partial x^2} = \frac{\phi(x_{i-1}, y_i, z_i) - 2\phi(x_i, y_i, z_i) + \phi(x_{i+1}, y_i, z_i)}{h^2} \tag{2}$$

$$\frac{\partial^2 \phi}{\partial y^2} = \frac{\phi(x_i, y_{i-1}, z_i) - 2\phi(x_i, y_i, z_i) + \phi(x_i, y_{i+1}, z_i)}{k^2} \tag{3}$$

$$\frac{\partial^2 \phi}{\partial z^2} = \frac{\phi(x_i, y_i, z_{i-1}) - 2\phi(x_i, y_i, z_i) + \phi(x_i, y_i, z_{i+1})}{l^2} \tag{4}$$

where h, k and l are the step sizes in the x, y and z directions respectively. Using the Laplace equation from (1) we have

$$\phi(x_i, y_i, z_i) = \frac{\phi(x_{i+1}, y_i, z_i) + \phi(x_{i-1}, y_i, z_i)}{6h^2}$$
$$+ \frac{\phi(x_i, y_{i-1}, z_i) + \phi(x_i, y_{i+1}, z_i)}{6k^2} + \frac{\phi(x_i, y_i, z_{i-1}) + \phi(x_i, y_i, z_{i+1})}{6l^2}$$

The above potential values are computed until the maximum difference between two successive iterations is below a certain threshold ζ. Generally, ζ is chosen to be 10^{-12}.

4.3 Computing Heat-Flow Lines

Streamlines or the heat flow lines are orthogonal to the isothermal (equipotential) surfaces. Each of the streamlines starts from the boundary points on the brain surface and progresses towards the designated shapecenter. Each of these streamlines approaches the shapecenter at unique angle(s), which remain constant along the streamline. This property is endowed by construction. The streamlines are computed by solving the following differential equation,

$$\frac{\partial X}{\partial t} = -\eta \nabla \phi[X(t)] \tag{5}$$

where $X = [x, y, z]^T$ is the coordinate vector and η is the normalization constant. MATLAB's (version R2014b) ode23 routine is used to solve the system of differential equations. The differential equation solver requires the potential values at the non-grid points within the domain U. The intermediate values are interpolated from the neighboring grid points using a local bilinear fitting model as,

$$\phi(x, y, z) = p_1 xyz + p_2 xy + p_3 yz + p_4 zx + p_5 x + p_6 y + p_7 z + p_8 \tag{6}$$

where $p_i's$ are constants. Eight neighborhood grid points are used to calculate the $p_i's$ and these are used to interpolate the ϕ at a non-grid point using the above equation.

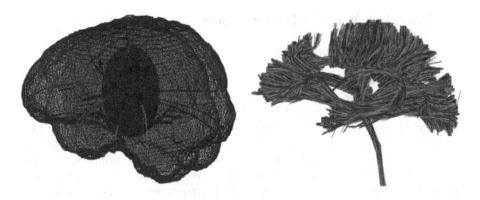

Heat-flow lines and Isosurfaces   Fiber tract bundle

Fig. 1. Left: 3D view of different equipotential surfaces are shown. The heat-flow lines emanating from the surface approach the shapecenter at unique polar and azimuthal angles. These angles remain constant along the streamlines. Intersect the surfaces at right angles. **Right:** The white matter fibers to be classified into different groups.

4.4 Parameterizing the Brain

Each streamline originating from each of the boundary points approaches the shapecenter at a unique angle. These angles remain constant along the streamlines. In case of three dimensional objects the angle of approach is characterized by the elevation (θ) and the azimuthal (ψ) angles. The vector between the shapecenter and the end point of the streamline is calculated. The angles are calculated using the Cartesian to spherical coordinate transformation

$$\psi = \text{atan2}(y, x); \quad \theta = \text{atan2}(\sqrt{x^2 + y^2}, z) \tag{7}$$

The streamlines intersect the equipotential surfaces at right angles (see Fig. 1). Each point of intersection generates a tuple $[\phi, \theta, \psi]^T$ for the corresponding Cartesian coordinates $[x, y, z]^T$.

5 Mapping the White Matter Fibers

After the whole brain is parameterized as mentioned above, each fiber tract is mapped to the new coordinate system, i.e., in the spherical space. At this stage, we have a bijective mapping between the Cartesian coordinates of every voxel in the brain and the newly computed coordinate system. A KD-tree structure is built using the native brain coordinates for ϕ, θ and ψ. For every point on the fiber streamline, the algorithm searches for ten neighborhood points and computes a weighted average to get the corresponding coordinate in the target domain. This process establishes the mapping of fibers in the target domain.

6 Clustering White Matter Fibers

6.1 Tracking White Matter Fibers

Data was obtained from Alzheimer's Disease Neuorimaging Initiative for the Department of Defense (ADNI-DoD). For each of the DTI images, 46 volumes were acquired with 5 T2 weighted B0 volumes and 41 diffusion-weighted volumes with voxel size of $1.36 \times 1.36 \times 2.7\,\text{mm}^3$. The scans were acquired using a GE 3.0T scanner, using echo planar imaging with parameters: $TR/TE = 9050/62\,\text{ms}$. Images were corrected for eddy-current distortions and skull-stripped. The diffusion gradient vectors are rotated based on the matrix transformation resulting from eddy-current correction. Whole-brain tractography was performed with Camino (http://cmic.cs.ucl.ac.uk/camino/), an open source software package that uses either streamline or probabilistic methods to reconstruct fiber paths. We performed fiber a probabilistic algorithm, called the 'Probabilistic Index of Connectivity' (PICo) in Camino [15]. Seed points were chosen at those voxels whose FA values were greater than 0.2. Monte Carlo simulation was used to generate fibers proceeding from the seed points throughout the entire brain [16]. Streamline fiber tracing followed the voxel-wise PDF profile with the Euler interpolation method for 7 iterations per each seed point. The maximum fiber turning angle was set to 60 degree/voxel, and tracing stopped at any voxel whose FA was less than 0.2.

For the purpose of comparison against the ground truth, manual labeling was performed by experts in neuroanatomy. Essentially, the FA images of these subjects were registered to a single-subject template in the ICBM-152 space called the "Type II Eve Atlas" (a 32-year-old healthy female) [17]. The entire brain of the "Eve" template was parcellated using 130 bilateral ROIs [18]. The labeled template ROIs were re-assigned to both subjects by warping them with the deformation fields generated by Advanced Neuroimaging Tools (ANTs) [19]. Each tract was manually edited to remove visible outliers. For each tract, there is a certain set of ROIs that it is intersects – a fiber must traverse all the required ROIs for a given tract to be considered, otherwise the fiber was discarded.

6.2 Unsupervised Clustering of White Matter Fibers

Various atlas based fiber clustering techniques are being used widely [20,21]. However, in our knowledge a completely automated fiber clustering method is non-existent. The authors in [11] claim that the presented method is automatic. However, the method requires manual region of interest labeling for seeding the fiber tractography algorithms. Manual delineation can be a time consuming and laborious process, and does not provide a fully automated method. Furthermore, the robustness of the clustering algorithm under a whole brain tractography can be variabled depending on the skill and expertise of the labeler.

Spectral Clustering is one of the widely used unsupervised clustering methods. The details of the method are available in [22,23]. A spectral clustering method requires a similarity criterion (or a distance metric) to be defined. This distance metric is used to compare all the N fibers with each other to create the affinity matrix of size $N \times N$. The idea behind spectral clustering is to approximate the affinity matrix based on its largest eigenvalues. If k eigenvalues are chosen, it implies that the data is distributed in a space spanned by the corresponding k eigenvectors. Here we choose k as the same as expected number of clusters.

Before clustering can be performed on the white matter tracts, the fiber tracts need to pre-processed. These pre-processing steps are crucial for good clustering results. All the white matter fibers are reparameterized using the arc length to contain the same number of points. The resampled tracks are mapped into the spherical domain as mentioned in Sect. 5. At this point, for each Cartesian coordinate $[x, y, z]$ on the track we have an equivalent coordinate $[\phi, \theta, \psi]$ in the spherical domain. The distance metric (d_{ij}) used for constructing the affinity matrix is defined as sum of squared differences on the new mapped coordinates. Thus, if i and j are two fibers and N is the total number of points in a track.

$$d_{ij} = \sum_{k=1}^{N}(p_i^k - p_j^k)^2$$

where p_i^k is one of the coordinates, i.e., ϕ, θ or ψ of the kth point in the fiber i. The hierarchical clustering is performed in this set of parameterized coordinates. The steps involved are enumerated as follows:

1. The mid-sagittal plane is located using the fractional anisotropy (FA) image and the white matter fibers are separated into the left and right hemispheres.
2. Corpus callosum is contained in both the hemispheres. Thus, it can be segmented by performing a logical AND operation on the two sets of fiber tracks obtained in the previous step.
3. An estimated desired number of clusters is provided by the user.
4. Spectral clustering is performed on ϕ coordinates of the tracks.
5. The mean variance of each of the clusters obtained is calculated. It is understood that if a group contains only one cluster, the mean variance will be low (typically <40).
6. The clusters with variance above the desired threshold is inspected and spectral clustering is performed again using the azimuthal angles (θ) of the tracks.
7. The previous step is repeated again and if there are mis-classified tracks another clustering is performed using the elevation angle ψ.
8. Because of the hierarchical nature of the clustering, we will generally end up with over-classification, i.e., we get more groups of fibers than desired.
9. The over classified clusters are merged. Each cluster is merged with those of the remaining ones and the resulting variance is calculated. If the variance is lower than the threshold, the clusters are merged. The process continues as long as there are more clusters than desired by the user.

The steps 4–7 in the algorithm is schematically represented in Fig. 2. Similar process is repeated for the right hemisphere.

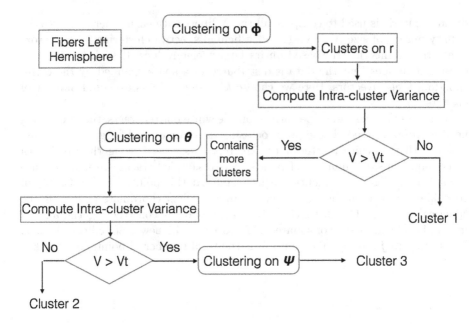

Fig. 2. The different steps in the hierarchical clustering process (steps 4–7) are shown. V represents the mean intra-cluster variance and Vt represents the variance threshold. Cluster 1, 2 and 3 represents the clusters obtained at each step of the process.

6.3   Results of Clustering

In Fig. 3, we show the results of the proposed hierarchical clustering. The left column shows the results of first level of clustering, i.e., with r co-ordinate. The tracks are overlayed on the corresponding FA image for anatomical reference. The variance of the cluster is mentioned below each panel. As expected, we found that the variance of the clusters containing a single group is comparatively lower than the ones which contained more than one groups. The groups with variance higher than 40 (threshold) were re-clustered as shown but with different coordinates until the variance is lower than the variance threshold. At this point we do have more sub-clusters than expected. We follow an agglomerative approach for combining the redundant clusters. The hierarchical nature of the method makes the clustering process tractable. For the purpose of validation, a ground truth data set was generated using manual labeling. A comparison between the proposed clustering method and the traditional spectral clustering method using Hausdroff distance as metric is shown. When compared to the ground truth the proposed method is able to retrieve all the fiber bundles as see in Fig. 4.

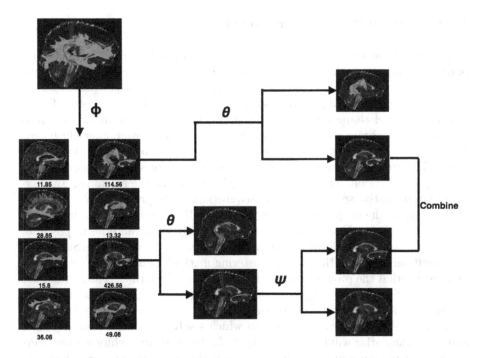

Fig. 3. The left column shows the result of clustering based on the ϕ coordinate. In the second column, two of the fiber bundles can be further classified. A second and third level of clustering is performed based of the azimuthal θ and polar ψ angles. At this stage, we have some over classified bundles as seen in the last column. The bundles with the combined variance less than a user defined threshold are combined.

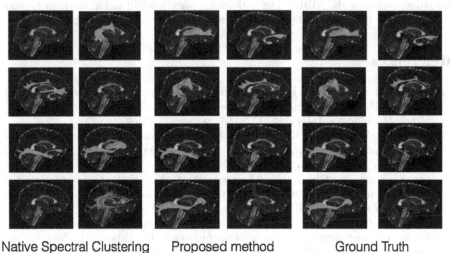

Native Spectral Clustering   Proposed method   Ground Truth

Fig. 4. A comparison between the clustering methods. The manual segmentation is shown in the right most column. The left and the right columns show spectral clustering using the Hausdroff distance and the proposed method respectively.

7   Conclusion and Future Work

In this paper we proposed a novel volumetric parameterization technique for parameterizing the brain to a sphere. Unlike prior methods which generally rely on surface parameterization, the method presented in this paper parameterizes the whole brain, following early work by [10]. This method may be useful for developing novel shape based-registration methods, mapping regions of interest, performing brain connectivity analysis and white matter fiber clustering. We have also shown a potential use of the method in clustering white matter tracts. The presented clustering method does not require any ROI based seeding or image registration. The fiber tractography as well as the clustering was performed in the native space of diffusion acquisition. In the present implementation of the method the shape-center is chosen manually. However, in the future the shapecenter can be chosen automatically, preferably at the anterior or posterior commissure and can be located automatically using tools such as FreeSurfer. We compared our results with spectral clustering methods using Hausdroff distance and showed that the proposed method out-performs the former. The method has to be tested for robustness against noisy data. In the future, we would like to use the method for statistical analysis on large datasets for comparing fiber tract geometries. We believe that, a method which solely relies on the subject data and not on any atlas will be particularly useful for clustering white matter fibers for surgical purposes and in subject with significant white matter deformities that cannot be represented in the white matter atlas.

Acknowledgements. This study was supported in part by a Consortium grant (U54 EB020403) from the NIH Institutes contributing to the Big Data to Knowledge (BD2K) Initiative, including the NIBIB. The authors are also thankful to Dr. Ratnesh Kumar from Teradeep Inc., Sunnyvale (California) for valuable insights and suggestions.

References

1. Floater, M.S., Hormann, K.: Surface parameterization: a tutorial and survey. In: Dodgson, N., Floater, M.S., Sabin, M. (eds.) Advances in Multiresolution for Geometric Modelling, vol. 1(1), pp. 157–186. Springer, Heidelberg (2005)
2. Gupta, V., Voruganti, H.K., Dasgupta, B.: Domain mapping for volumetric parameterization using harmonic functions. Comput. Aided Des. Appl. **11**(4), 426–435 (2014)
3. Gu, X., Wang, Y., Chan, T.F., Thompson, P.M., Yau, S.-T.: Genus zero surface conformal mapping and its application to brain surface mapping. IEEE Trans. Med. Imaging **23**(8), 949–958 (2004)
4. Wang, Y., Gu, X., Chan, T.F., Thompson, P.M., Yau, S.-T.: Brain surface conformal parameterization with algebraic functions. In: Larsen, R., Nielsen, M., Sporring, J. (eds.) MICCAI 2006. LNCS, vol. 4191, pp. 946–954. Springer, Heidelberg (2006). doi:10.1007/11866763_116
5. Wang, Y., Shi, J., Yin, X., Gu, X., Chan, T.F., Yau, S.-T., Toga, A.W., Thompson, P.M.: Brain surface conformal parameterization with the Ricci flow. IEEE Trans. Med. Imaging **31**(2), 251–264 (2012)

6. Mémoli, F., Sapiro, G., Osher, S.: Solving variational problems and partial differential equations mapping into general target manifolds. J. Comput. Phys. **195**(1), 263–292 (2004)

7. Gutman, B.A., Madsen, S.K., Toga, A.W., Thompson, P.M.: A family of fast spherical registration algorithms for cortical shapes. In: Shen, L., Liu, T., Yap, P.-T., Huang, H., Shen, D., Westin, C.-F. (eds.) MBIA 2013. LNCS, vol. 8159, pp. 246–257. Springer, Heidelberg (2013). doi:10.1007/978-3-319-02126-3_24

8. Shi, Y., Lai, R., Toga, A.W.: Conformal mapping via metric optimization with application for cortical label fusion. In: Gee, J.C., Joshi, S., Pohl, K.M., Wells, W.M., Zöllei, L. (eds.) IPMI 2013. LNCS, vol. 7917, pp. 244–255. Springer, Heidelberg (2013). doi:10.1007/978-3-642-38868-2_21

9. Lombaert, H., Arcaro, M., Ayache, N.: Brain transfer: spectral analysis of cortical surfaces and functional maps. In: Ourselin, S., Alexander, D.C., Westin, C.-F., Cardoso, M.J. (eds.) IPMI 2015. LNCS, vol. 9123, pp. 474–487. Springer, Heidelberg (2015). doi:10.1007/978-3-319-19992-4_37

10. Wang, Y., Gu, X., Chan, T.F., Thompson, P.M., Yau, S.T.: Volumetric harmonic brain mapping. In: IEEE International Symposium on Biomedical Imaging: Nano to Macro, pp. 1275–1278. IEEE (2004)

11. O'Donnell, L., Kubicki, M., Shenton, M.E., Dreusicke, M.H., Grimson, W.E.L., Westin, C.F.: A method for clustering white matter fiber tracts. Am. J. Neuroradiol. **27**(5), 1032–1036 (2006)

12. Corouge, I., Gouttard, S., Gerig, G.: Towards a shape model of white matter fiber bundles using diffusion tensor MRI. In: IEEE International Symposium on Biomedical Imaging: Nano to Macro. pp. 344–347. IEEE (2004)

13. Liu, M., Vemuri, B.C., Deriche, R.: Unsupervised automatic white matter fiber clustering using a Gaussian mixture model. In: 2012 9th IEEE International Symposium on Biomedical Imaging (ISBI), pp. 522–525. IEEE (2012)

14. Guevara, P., Poupon, C., Rivière, D., Cointepas, Y., Descoteaux, M., Thirion, B., Mangin, J.F.: Robust clustering of massive tractography datasets. NeuroImage **54**(3), 1975–1993 (2011)

15. Cook, P., Bai, Y., Nedjati-Gilani, S., Seunarine, K., Hall, M., Parker, G., Alexander, D.: Camino: open-source diffusion-MRI reconstruction and processing. In: 14th Scientific Meeting of the International Society for Magnetic Resonance in Medicine, Seattle, WA, USA, vol. 2759 (2006)

16. Parker, G.J.M., Alexander, D.C.: Probabilistic Monte Carlo based mapping of cerebral connections utilising whole-brain crossing fibre information. In: Taylor, C., Noble, J.A. (eds.) IPMI 2003. LNCS, vol. 2732, pp. 684–695. Springer, Heidelberg (2003). doi:10.1007/978-3-540-45087-0_57

17. Oishi, K., Faria, A., Jiang, H., Li, X., Akhter, K., Zhang, J., Hsu, J.T., Miller, M.I., van Zijl, P.C., Albert, M., Lyketsos, C.G., Woods, R., Toga, A.W., Pike, G.B., Rosa-Neto, P., Evans, A., Mazziotta, J., Mori, S.: Atlas-based whole brain white matter analysis using large deformation diffeomorphic metric mapping: application to normal elderly and Alzheimer's disease participants. NeuroImage **46**(2), 486–499 (2009)

18. Zhang, Y., Zhang, J., Oishi, K., Faria, A.V., Jiang, H., Li, X., Akhter, K., Rosa-Neto, P., Pike, G.B., Evans, A., et al.: Atlas-guided tract reconstruction for automated and comprehensive examination of the white matter anatomy. NeuroImage **52**(4), 1289–1301 (2010)

19. Avants, B.B., Epstein, C.L., Grossman, M., Gee, J.C.: Symmetric diffeomorphic image registration with cross-correlation: evaluating automated labeling of elderly and neurodegenerative brain. Med. Image Anal. **12**(1), 26–41 (2008)

20. O'Donnell, L.J., Westin, C.F.: Automatic tractography segmentation using a high-dimensional white matter atlas. IEEE Trans. Med. Imaging **26**(11), 1562–1575 (2007)
21. Jin, Y., Shi, Y., Zhan, L., Gutman, B.A., de Zubicaray, G.I., McMahon, K.L., Wright, M.J., Toga, A.W., Thompson, P.M.: Automatic clustering of white matter fibers in brain diffusion MRI with an application to genetics. NeuroImage **100**, 75–90 (2014)
22. Filippone, M., Camastra, F., Masulli, F., Rovetta, S.: A survey of kernel and spectral methods for clustering. Pattern Recogn. **41**(1), 176–190 (2008)
23. Von Luxburg, U.: A tutorial on spectral clustering. Stat. Comput. **17**(4), 395–416 (2007)

Deep Spectral-Based Shape Features
for Alzheimer's Disease Classification

Mahsa Shakeri[1,2]($\boxtimes$), Herve Lombaert[3], Shashank Tripathi[1],
Samuel Kadoury[1,2], and for the Alzheimer's Disease Neuroimaging Initiative

[1] Medical, Polytechnique Montreal, Montreal, Canada
mahsa.shakeri@polymtl.ca
[2] CHU Sainte-Justine Research Center, Montreal, Canada
[3] Inria Sophia-Antipolis, Valbonne, France

Abstract. Alzheimer's disease (AD) and mild cognitive impairment
(MCI) are the most prevalent neurodegenerative brain diseases in elderly
population. Recent studies on medical imaging and biological data have
shown morphological alterations of subcortical structures in patients
with these pathologies. In this work, we take advantage of these structural deformations for classification purposes. First, triangulated surface
meshes are extracted from segmented hippocampus structures in MRI
and point-to-point correspondences are established among population of
surfaces using a spectral matching method. Then, a deep learning variational auto-encoder is applied on the vertex coordinates of the mesh
models to learn the low dimensional feature representation. A multi-layer
perceptrons using softmax activation is trained simultaneously to classify Alzheimer's patients from normal subjects. Experiments on ADNI
dataset demonstrate the potential of the proposed method in classification of normal individuals from early MCI (EMCI), late MCI (LMCI),
and AD subjects with classification rates outperforming standard SVM
based approach.

Keywords: Classification · Spectral matching · Variational
autoencoder · Alzheimer's disease

1 Introduction

Alzheimer's disease (AD) is characterized by progressive impairment of cognitive
and memory functions in elderly population. Considering its worldwide preva-
lence, early diagnosis of this disease might have a huge impact on the overall
well-being of the population, and the burden to caregivers, as well as the associated financial costs to the world's health system. Studies reported that AD

Data used in preparation of this article were obtained from the Alzheimer's Disease
Neuroimaging Initiative (ADNI) database (adni.loni.usc.edu). As such, the investigators within the ADNI contributed to the design and implementation of ADNI
and/or provided data but did not participate in analysis or writing of this report.
A complete listing of ADNI investigators can be found at http://adni.loni.usc.edu/
wp-content/uploads/how_to_apply/ADNI_Acknowledgement_List.pdf.

© Springer International Publishing AG 2016
M. Reuter et al. (Eds.): SeSAMI 2016, LNCS 10126, pp. 15–24, 2016.
DOI: 10.1007/978-3-319-51237-2_2

can be diagnosed by clinical assessments in most of the cases [1], while by the time the patient is diagnosed the disease progression may have deteriorated. Therefore, early diagnosis of this neuropathology is of special interest.

Mild cognitive impairment (MCI) is considered as a transition state between normal aging and dementia [2]. The cognitive deficits in MCI patients are not as severe as those seen in individuals with AD. However, studies have suggested that about 10–12% of subjects with MCI progress to AD per year [2]. Therefore, these individuals with milder degrees of cognitive and functional impairment than AD patients are particularly interesting subjects, since biomarker manifestation could potentially be different at such an early stage of the disease.

Studies have shown that the neuropathological changes in AD and MCI affect the hippocampus structure, which is a brain region crucial to various cognitive functions [3]. Neuroimaging datasets for AD including magnetic resonance imaging (MRI) and other types of biomarkers have shown considerable promise to detect longitudinal changes in subjects [4], by offering rich information on the patients morphometric and anatomical profiles. Their use stems from the premise that morphological changes may be more reproducible and more precisely measured with MRI than other parameters such as clinical scores, cerebrospinal fluid (CSF), or proteomic assessments.

Recent advances in medical imaging and classification techniques have led to a better discrimination between Alzheimer's disease and healthy aging. Because of the high dimensionality of medical image, various dimensionality reduction approaches have been developed to facilitate and enhance classification accuracy. A simple method is principal components analysis (PCA) [5], which finds the directions of greatest variance in the dataset and represents each data point by its coordinates along each of these directions. A nonlinear generalization of PCA is multi-layer autoencoders (AE) [6], which is a feedforward neural network to encode the input into a more compact from and reconstruct the input with the learned representation. Among available AE architectures, the deep variational autoencoder (VAE) [7] method has recently become popular in computer vision due to its capability to learn a manifold without the assumption of linearity in addition to its generative property.

With respect to surface representation, recent studies have shown the advantage of spectral shape description compared to Euclidean surface representation [8–10]. The use of eigenvalues have led to interesting results for AD classification in [11], where Laplace-Beltrami spectrum on the intrinsic geometry of the structural meshes was computed to define the shape descriptors. The spectral coordinates, which were derived from the Laplacian eigenfunctions of shapes have been used in [8] to parametrize surfaces explicitly. The authors applied a Random Decision Forest classifier on spectral representation of surfaces and achieved a significant improvement on cortical parcellations. Also, in [9,10], the eigendecomposition of the surfaces in the spectral domain were used to provide pointwise information on meshes and establish accurate point-to-point correspondences across surfaces.

In this work, we present a surface-based classification technique based on classification of spectral features using variational stacked auto-encoders. We first extract 3D surface meshes of hippocampus structures from segmented binary MR images. Then, the point-to-point surface correspondences is established across populations (NC, AD, EMCI, LMCI) using a spectral matching approach. In spectral based shape matching approach, relationships are modeled as graphs and an eigendecomposition on these graphs enables us to match similar features. Once the matched surfaces are created, the vertex coordinates are used as shape feature descriptors. Then, variational autoencoder (VAE) obtains the non-linear low-dimensional embedding of the shape features. A multi-layer perceptron (MLP) classifier is simultaneously trained to model the non-linear decision boundaries between classes.

The work follows on the prior work of [12], which used a Stacked Auto-Encoder (SAE) to discover the latent representation from the grey matter (GM) tissue densities and voxel intensities. Unlike Suk and Shen [12], which selects intensity and volume based features from MRI and PET modalities, we create the feature descriptors from matched hippocampi surfaces extracted from MRI. Moreover, instead of training a separate classifier on the low dimensional features as in [12], we add a softmax multi-layer perceptron on top of our variational autoencoder network to obtain both dimensionality reduction and the classification output at the same time.

The rest of the paper is organized as follows. In Sect. 2, we present the morphological feature extraction method using spectral shape matching, as well as the feature representation and classification method based on variational autoencoder and multi-layer perceptron. Section 3 includes the description of the dataset, experiments and discussion. Our conclusions are presented in Sect. 4, along with envisioned future research directions.

2   Methodology

Given MR images along with their corresponding hippocampus segmentations (produced manually or automatically), we first extract features from MRI as explained in Sect. 2.1. Then, we use a deep variational autoencoder (VAE) to learn a latent feature representation from the low-level features and train a multi-layer perceptron (MLP) for classification purposes in Sect. 2.2.

2.1   Shape Feature Extraction Using Spectral Matching

Given a reference surface mesh S_r and a population of n surfaces $\{S_i\}_{i=1..n}$, the spectral matching between each surface meshe S_i and S_r is done in a two step process. First, an initial map is calculated between the two surfaces [9]. This initial map is then used in the second step to establish a smooth map between the two meshes [10].

Here, we consider vertices and neighbouring points in each surface mesh as nodes and edges of a graph. Then a laplacian graph is created for each surface graph from the set of vertices and edges of each mesh. The general Laplacian operator L_i [13] is defined on each surface as following:

$$L_i = G_i^{-1} (D_i - W_i) \tag{1}$$

where W_i is the weighted adjacency matrix, which is created based on a distance between connected nodes. The term D_i is a diagonal matrix, in which the elements are set by the degree of vertices. G_i is a node weighting matrix created based on the mean curvature at each node as described in [14].

The eigendecomposition of Laplacian matrix L_i provides its spectral components. After reordering the spectral components by finding the optimal permutation of components between the pair of meshes, regularization is performed by matching the spectral embeddings. The correspondence initial map c between each pair of vertices on S_i and S_r is established with a simple nearest-neighbour search between their spectral representations.

In the next step, given initial map c, the final smooth map between two surfaces S_i and S_r is obtained. In this process, an association graph is defined as the union of the set of vertices and edges of two surfaces with an initial set of correspondence links c between both surfaces. Then, a Laplacian matrix is created for the association graph, and the spectral decomposition is computed to produce a shared set of eigenvectors that enables a direct mapping between two meshes S_i and S_r.

Once all 3D meshes are matched to the reference, the vertices of all surfaces are rearranged to create the new reconstructed meshes with consistent vertex ordering. Now, the shape descriptor x_i will be created for the surface S_i as a vector of (X, Y, Z) coordinate of all vertices.

2.2   Feature Learning and Classification

In this work we use a deep learning-based feature representation method to improve the classification accuracy. Here, we take inspiration from the variational autoencoder network, which learns the low-dimensional manifold without the linearity assumption and has a generative model. In this section, we explain the proposed network architecture, which is a combination of a variational autoencoder network (VAE) and a softmax multi-layer perceptron (MLP). The combined VAE-MLP network architecture is shown in Fig. 1.

Deep Variational Autoencoder and MLP Classifier

Auto-encoders are a type of deep neural networks structurally defined by input, hidden, and output layers. Given the input data $x \in R^D$ defined from the spectral representation of mesh shapes, an auto-encoder maps it to a latent representation $z \in R^d$ (encoding), which could be used for unsupervised learning or for feature extraction. The representation z from the hidden layer is then mapped back to a vector $y \in R^D$ (decoding), which approximately reconstructs the input vector x. The hidden layer in the middle, i.e., z, can be constrained to be a bottleneck to learn compact representations of the input data.

Variational autoencoder (VAE) assumes that data is generated by a directed graphical model with a latent variable z. VAE uses the encoder network to map the input x into the continuous latent variables ($q_\phi(z|x)$) and uses decoder network to map latent variables to reconstructed data ($p_\theta(x|z)$), where ϕ and θ are the parameters of the encoder (recognition model) and decoder (generative model), respectively.

The lower bound VAE loss function of the variational autoencoder for individual datapoint x_i has the following form:

$$L_{VAE}(\theta, \phi; x_i) = -D_{KL}\left(q_\phi\left(z|x_i\right)||p_\theta\left(z\right)\right) + E_{q_\phi(z|x_i)}\left[\log p_\theta\left(x_i|z\right)\right] \quad (2)$$

The first component is the regularization term, which is the KL divergence of the approximate posterior from the prior, while the second term is the expected reconstruction error. As shown in [7], we assume both $p_\theta\left(z\right)$ and $q_\phi\left(z|x_i\right)$ as Gaussian. Given J as the dimensionality of z and K as the number of samples per datapoint, the resulting estimator for x_i will be as follows:

$$L_{VAE}(\theta, \phi; x_i) = -\frac{1}{2}\sum_{j=1}^{J}\left(1 + \log\left(\sigma_j^2\right) - \mu_j^2 - \sigma_j^2\right) + \frac{1}{K}\sum_{k=1}^{K}\log p_\theta\left(x_i|z_{i,k}\right) \quad (3)$$

where, $z_{i,k} = \mu_i + \sigma_i \odot \epsilon_k$ and $\epsilon_k \sim N\left(0, I\right)$.

Here, μ and σ can be computed using the deterministic encoder network. The reconstruction (decoding) term of $\log p_\theta\left(x_i|z_{i,k}\right)$ could be set as a Bernoulli cross-entropy loss function.

The low dimensional features $z_i = \mu_i + \sigma_i$ from the latent layer are fed to an MLP classifier for solving the classification problem. For the last layer, we use the cross entropy loss function and the softmax activation function, which is standard for classification problems [15]. The softmax function ensures that the network outputs are all between zero and one, and that they sum to one on every time step. Therefore, they can be interpreted as the posterior probabilities, given all the inputs up to the current one. We set the number of units in the classification output layer to be equal to the number of classes of interest (i.e., two).

The Network Architecture

Annotated medical image datasets tend to be small and generally hard to obtain. This increases the risk of network overfitting in medical applications. Therefore, we make a series of design choices for our network to avoid overfitting. Our network includes L_2 regularization at each layer to penalize the squared magnitude of all parameters directly in the objective function. That is, for every weight w in the network, we add the term $\frac{1}{2}\lambda w^2$ to the cost function, where λ is the regularization strength.

We also add a drop out layer with the probability of 0.5 after each dense layer. During training, dropout is implemented by only keeping a neurone active with some probability p, or setting it to zero otherwise. Network weights are set based on the uniform initialization scaled by the square root of the number of inputs.

We train the network for 100 epochs with batch size of 28 starting with a learning rate of 0.00001 and dropping it at a logarithmic rate to 0.000001. For the deep learning library, we use Keras and Theano. We determine the number of hidden units based on the classification results. The optimal structure of the network is shown in Fig. 1.

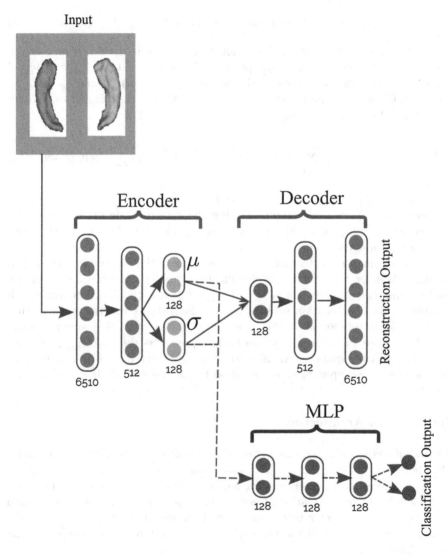

Fig. 1. The architecture of our proposed network. The numbers mentioned under each layer correspond to the layer's dimension.

3 Experiments

We evaluate the performance of our approach on a popular brain imaging dataset in Alzheimer's disease, namely the Alzheimer's Disease Neuroimaging Initiative (ADNI). The ADNI database (adni.loni.usc.edu) was launched in 2003 as a public-private partnership, led by Principal Investigator Michael W. Weiner, MD. The primary goal of ADNI has been to test whether serial magnetic resonance imaging (MRI), positron emission tomography (PET), other biological markers, and clinical and neuropsychological assessment can be combined to measure the progression of mild cognitive impairment (MCI) and early Alzheimer's disease (AD). For up-to-date information, see www.adni-info.org. The database of ADNI consists of cross-sectional and longitudinal data including 1.5 or 3.0 T structural MR images. The detailed description of the MRI protocol of ADNI is provided in [16].

For this study, a subset of latest 1.5 T MR images is used including 150 normal controls (NC), 90 AD patients, 160 early MCI (EMCI), and 160 individuals with late MCI (LMCI). ADNI performed additional post-processing steps on MR images to correct certain image artifacts and to enhance standardization across sites and platforms [16]. The post-processing steps include gradient nonlinearity correction, intensity inhomogeneity correction, bias field correction, and phantom-based geometrical scaling to remove calibration errors. In this work, we use these processed images. Here, hippocampi was segmented using FSL-FIRST automatic segmentation software package [17] and visual inspection was performed on the output binary masks to ensure the quality of the automatic segmentation.

Here we consider six binary classification problems: AD vs. NC, NC vs. EMCI, NC vs. LMCI, AD vs. EMCI, AD vs. LMCI, and EMCI vs. LMCI. We consider 20% of data for test and the rest for train. Each time 20% of train set is left out and used for validation. The whole process is repeated five times for unbiased evaluation. The regularization strength λ is set as 0.05 based on experimental results.

We tested different network architectures and realized that going deeper than the proposed model in Fig. 1 would not help improving the classification accuracy, however the dimensionality of the hidden and the latent unit had direct effect on the classification performance.

In the analysis of the results, the performance of the classifier are measured by its sensitivity (SE), specificity (SP) and accuracy (AC). Sensitivity, which is the ability of the classifier to correctly identify positive results, is defined as $TP/(TP+FN)$. Specificity refers to the ability to correctly identify negative results and is formulated as $TN/(FP+TN)$. Accuracy is defined as $(TP+TN)/(TP+TN+FN+FP)$.

As baseline, we train a linear Support Vector Machines (SVM) on the same dataset after applying principle components analysis (PCA) for dimensionality reduction. The features are extracted from 3D surface meshes after applying spectral matching in the same way as our proposed method. The classification accuracy for the proposed and the baseline methods is illustrated in Fig. 2. We

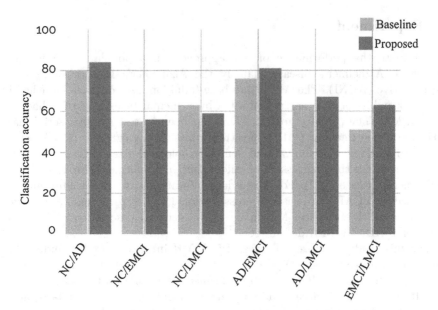

Fig. 2. Comparison of the classification accuracy with a baseline approach using the same spectral-based shape feature representation. The VAE-based method achieved higher accuracy in most of the cases.

summarize the classification accuracy along with the sensitivity (SE), and specificity (SP) measures in Table 1.

These results show that our method produces higher accuracy in most of the cases. As expected, the best classification accuracies are those obtained for groups, which are well separated diagnostically. For instance, 84% and 81% for the classification of NC versus AD and EMCI versus AD, respectively. The computational time of both methods is around 60 s for training on 300 surfaces and less than 5 ms for testing on one surface.

In addition, the obtained results is comparable to the previously proposed approaches that have used MRI based features. For instance, Suk and Shen [12] and Goryawala et al. [18] found the accuracy of 85% and 84%, respectively for the classification of NC versus AD. These method have also included additional information from PET modality or neuropsychological test to improve the classification performance. One future direction of our proposed approach would be to include a combination of informative features to reach a higher accuracy.

Table 1. Comparison of the classification accuracy (AC%), sensitivity (SE%), and specificity (SP%) with a baseline method using the same spectral-based shape feature descriptor. The proposed method achieved higher accuracy in most of the cases.

	NC/AD			NC/EMCI			NC/LMCI			AD/EMCI			AD/LMCI			EMCI/LMCI		
	AC	SE	SP	AC	SE	SP	AC	SE	SP	AC	SE	SP	AC	SE	SP	AC	SE	SP
Baseline	80	70	86	55	52	58	**63**	**56**	**75**	76	65	71	63	58	66	51	50	52
Proposed	**84**	**73**	**89**	**56**	**52**	**60**	59	52	64	**81**	**70**	**82**	**67**	**58**	**73**	**63**	**62**	**66**

4   Conclusions

In this paper we have proposed a deep learning method based on a spectral feature representation using hippocampus morphology for the classification of Alzheimer's Disease. The morphological features were extracted as 3D surface meshes from MR image and spectral matching process was used to establish point-to-point correspondences in mesh vertices. A variational autoencoder was trained to find the latent feature representation from hippocampus morphological variations. A softmax classifier was applied to differentiate between NC, EMCI, LMCI, and AD.

Experimental evaluation on the ADNI dataset demonstrates the effectiveness of our approach especially in classifying AD vs. NC and AD vs. EMCI. This work shows the importance of the VAE-based morphological feature representation in improving the diagnosis accuracy in different stages of dementia. Future research directions include adding other informative features, such as cognitive information and multimodal data (e.g., PET) to increase the classification accuracy.

Acknowledgements. Funding was provided by the Canada Research Chairs and from the CHU Sainte-Justine Hospital's Research Center, Montreal, Canada.

ADNI data collection and sharing for this project was funded by the Alzheimer's Disease Neuroimaging Initiative (ADNI) (National Institutes of Health Grant U01 AG024904) and DOD ADNI (Department of Defense award number W81XWH-12-2-0012). ADNI is funded by the National Institute on Aging, the National Institute of Biomedical Imaging and Bioengineering, and through generous contributions from the following: AbbVie, Alzheimer's Association; Alzheimer's Drug Discovery Foundation; Araclon Biotech; BioClinica, Inc.; Biogen; Bristol-Myers Squibb Company; CereSpir, Inc.; Eisai Inc.; Elan Pharmaceuticals, Inc.; Eli Lilly and Company; EuroImmun; F. Hoffmann-La Roche Ltd and its affiliated company Genentech, Inc.; Fujirebio; GE Healthcare; IXICO Ltd.; Janssen Alzheimer Immunotherapy Research & Development, LLC.; Johnson & Johnson Pharmaceutical Research & Development LLC.; Lumosity; Lundbeck; Merck & Co., Inc.; Meso Scale Diagnostics, LLC.; NeuroRx Research; Neurotrack Technologies; Novartis Pharmaceuticals Corporation; Pfizer Inc.; Piramal Imaging; Servier; Takeda Pharmaceutical Company; and Transition Therapeutics. The Canadian Institutes of Health Research is providing funds to support ADNI clinical sites in Canada. Private sector contributions are facilitated by the Foundation for the National Institutes of Health (www.fnih.org). The grantee organization is the Northern California Institute for Research and Education, and the study is coordinated by the Alzheimer's Disease Cooperative Study at the University of California, San Diego. ADNI data are disseminated by the Laboratory for Neuro Imaging at the University of Southern California.

References

1. Ranginwala, N.A., Hynan, L.S., Weiner, M.F., White, C.L.I.: Clinical criteria for the diagnosis of Alzheimer disease: still good after all these years. Am. J. Geriatr. Psychiatry **16**(5), 384–388 (2008)

2. Petersen, R., Smith, G., Waring, S., Ivnik, R., Tangalos, E., Kokmen, E.: Mild cognitive impairment: clinical characterization and outcome. Arch. Neurol. **56**(3), 303–308 (1999)
3. Du, A.T., Schuff, N., et al.: Magnetic resonance imaging of the entorhinal cortex and hippocampus in mild cognitive impairment and Alzheimer's disease. J. Neurol. Neurosurg. Psychiatry **71**, 441–447 (2001)
4. Wyman, B., Harvey, D., Crawford, K., Bernstein, M., Carmichael, O., Cole, P., Crane, P., Decarli, C., Fox, N., Gunter, J., Hill, D., Killiany, R., Pachai, C., Schwarz, A., Schuff, N., Senjem, M., Suhy, J., Thompson, P., Weiner, M., Jack, C.: Standardization of analysis sets for reporting results from ADNI MRI data. Alzheimer's Dement. **9**(3), 332–337 (2013)
5. Davatzikos, C., Fan, Y., Wu, X., Shen, D., Resnick, S.: Alzheimer's disease via pattern classification of MRI. Neurobiol. Aging **29**(4), 514–523 (2008)
6. Bengio, Y.: Learning deep architectures for AI. Found. Trends Mach. Learn. **2**(1), 1–127 (2009)
7. Kingma, D.P., Welling, M.: Auto-encoding variational Bayes. In: International Conference on Learning Representations (ICLR) (2013)
8. Lombaert, H., Criminisi, A., Ayache, N.: Spectral forests: learning of surface data, application to cortical parcellation. In: Navab, N., Hornegger, J., Wells, W.M., Frangi, A.F. (eds.) MICCAI 2015. LNCS, vol. 9349, pp. 547–555. Springer, Heidelberg (2015). doi:10.1007/978-3-319-24553-9_67
9. Lombaert, H., Grady, L., Polimeni, J.R., Cheriet, F.: FOCUSR: feature oriented correspondence using spectral regularization – a method for precise surface matching. IEEE Trans. Pattern Anal. Mach. Intell. **35**(9), 2143–2160 (2013)
10. Lombaert, H., Sporring, J., Siddiqi, K.: Diffeomorphic spectral matching of cortical surfaces. In: Gee, J.C., Joshi, S., Pohl, K.M., Wells, W.M., Zöllei, L. (eds.) IPMI 2013. LNCS, vol. 7917, pp. 376–389. Springer, Heidelberg (2013). doi:10.1007/978-3-642-38868-2_32
11. Wachinger, C., Reuter, M.: Domain adaptation for Alzheimer's disease diagnostics. NeuroImage **139**, 470–479 (2016)
12. Suk, H.-I., Shen, D.: Deep learning-based feature representation for AD/MCI classification. In: Mori, K., Sakuma, I., Sato, Y., Barillot, C., Navab, N. (eds.) MICCAI 2013. LNCS, vol. 8150, pp. 583–590. Springer, Heidelberg (2013). doi:10.1007/978-3-642-40763-5_72
13. Grady, L.J., Polimeni, J.R.: Discrete Calculus. Springer, Heidelberg (2010)
14. Shakeri, M., Lombaert, H., Datta, A.N., Oser, N., Ltourneau-Guillon, L., Lapointe, L.V., Martin, F., Malfait, D., Tucholka, A., Lippe, S., Kadoury, S.: Statistical shape analysis of subcortical structures using spectral matching. Comput. Med. Imaging Graph. **52**, 58–71 (2016)
15. Bishop, C.M.: Neural Networks for Pattern Recognition. Oxford University Press, Inc., New York (1995)
16. Jack, C., Bernstein, M., Fox, N., et al.: The Alzheimer's disease neuroimaging initiative (ADNI): MRI methods. J. Magn. Reson. Imaging: JMRI **27**(4), 685–691 (2008)
17. Patenaude, B., Smith, S.M., Kennedy, D.N., Jenkinson, M.: A Bayesian model of shape and appearance for subcortical brain segmentation. NeuroImage **56**, 907–922 (2011)
18. Goryawala, M., et al.: Inclusion of neuropsychological scores in atrophy models improves diagnostic classification of Alzheimer's disease and mild cognitive impairment. Comput. Intell. Neurosci. **2015**, 56 (2015)

Functional Maps for Brain Classification on Spectral Domain

Simone Melzi[1]([✉]), Alessandro Mella[1], Letizia Squarcina[2], Marcella Bellani[3],
Cinzia Perlini[4], Mirella Ruggeri[3], Carlo Alfredo Altamura[5], Paolo Brambilla[5,6],
and Umberto Castellani[1]

[1] Computer Science, University of Verona, Verona, Italy
simone.melzi@univr.it
[2] Scientific Institute IRCCS E. Medea, Bosisio Parini, Italy
[3] Section of Psychiatry, AOUI Verona, Verona, Italy
[4] Section of Clinical Psychology, Department of Neuroscience,
Biomedicine and Movement Sciences, University of Verona, Verona, Italy
[5] Department of Neurosciences and Mental Health, Fondazione IRCCS Ca Granda
Ospedale Maggiore Policlinico, University of Milan, Milan, Italy
[6] Department of Psychiatry and Behavioural Sciences,
University of Texas Health Science Center, Houston, TX, USA

Abstract. In this paper we exploit the Functional maps approach for brain classification. The functional representation of brain shapes, or their subparts, enables us to improve the detection of morphological abnormalities associated with the analyzed disease. The proposed method is based on the spectral shape paradigm that is largely used for generic geometric processing but still few exploited in the medical context. The key aspect of the Functional maps framework is that it moves the estimation of correspondences from the shape space to the functional space enhancing the potential of spectral analysis. Moreover, we propose a new kernel, called the Functional maps kernel (FM-kernel) for the Support Vector Machine (SVM) classification that is specifically designed to work on the functional space. The obtained results for bipolar disorder detection on the *putamen* regions are promising in comparison with other spectral-based approaches.

Keywords: Spectral shape analysis · Functional maps · Brain classification · Diseases and disorders detection

1 Introduction

Automatically detection of abnormal anatomical shapes derived from diseased subjects is a fundamental goal in medical imaging. This task is typically formulated as a two-class classification problem, assigning to each shape a healthy or diseased label [30,31]. In particular, thanks to the increased amount of data available, the attention of researchers is often focused on advanced learning-by-example methods [2,4,6,14,15,29]. These tools require good shape representation and measure that encodes the relationship between the shapes. The

© Springer International Publishing AG 2016
M. Reuter et al. (Eds.): SeSAMI 2016, LNCS 10126, pp. 25–36, 2016.
DOI: 10.1007/978-3-319-51237-2_3

desired representation should be informative, concise and efficient in computational terms. In order to capture possible brain deformations due to the disease, it is convenient to exploit geometry and topology properties of the anatomical parts as shape representation [12,13,18]. To this aim, new spectral shape descriptors and methods have been adopted in this area [5,26], aiming at investigating advanced shape analysis approaches for the characterization of brain structures.

In this work we propose a new method for shape classification based on the Functional maps framework [22]. The main idea of Functional maps consists of defining a functional space for each surface and therefore representing relations between surfaces as linear maps between these functional spaces. In this fashion, the correspondences between pair of shapes is carried out on the functional representation rather than the physical space in a more flexible and easy to compute way. The characterizations of the shapes are based on point descriptors and parts derived from a shape segmentation procedure that can be encoded as functions defined on the surfaces. These corresponding functions give rise to linear constraints on the linear map between the two spaces. The solution can be computed by solving an optimization problem. Finally, choosing a proper basis for each functional space, the desired Functional maps can be carried out by applying standard linear algebraic techniques.

The contribution of the proposed method is two-fold:

- Firstly we extend the use of Functional map to the medical domain, to improve the encoding of morphological relations between pairs of brain-shapes.
- Secondly we propose a new dissimilarity measure properly designed for the functional space. In particular, from this dissimilarity measure we derived a well defined new kernel, namely the Functional maps kernel (FM-Kernel) that is effective and theoretically founded.

We evaluated our method for the characterization of brain abnormalities in the context of mental health research. In particular, we propose a brain classification study on a dataset of patients affected by bipolar disorder and healthy controls. We focused on the *putamen* region, which is a deep gray matter brain structure, part of the basal ganglia, a functional and anatomical heterogeneous region which is thought to be affected, particularly in shape, by bipolar disorder [17]. In order to check the actual effectiveness of the proposed method and the richness added by the Functional maps framework in this context, we compared our method with more classical shape analysis methods based on a spectral approach.

Roadmap. The rest of the paper is organized as follows. In Sect. 2 we give a brief overview of the related works, highlighting connections with our method. Section 3 summarizes the background on the Functional maps framework. The proposed method and the derived FM-Kernel are presented in Sect. 4. Then, the experimental Sect. 5 shows the results of our approach in comparison with other spectral-based methods for the brain classification on the putamen regions. Finally, in Sect. 6, some conclusions are drawn and future works are envisaged.

2   Related Work

In literature there are plenty of methods for identifying and detecting alterations in anatomical shapes. For brevity here we focus on the approaches that characterize the shapes by adopting a spectral shape analysis strategy. A first method based on spectral properties was proposed in [11], where spherical harmonic descriptors (SPHARM) are computed on brain surfaces after a shapes registration step. In [26] Reuter et al. introduced a spectral global descriptor, namely *Shape-DNA*. This signature is defined as the increasing ordered sequence of the first Laplace-Beltrami operator (LBO) eigenvalues. The Shape-DNA is invariant to the isometric deformations and by neglecting higher frequencies of the shape it is also robust to noise. This descriptor is proposed for two different versions: the external surfaces and the entire volume. The two surface-based and volume-based versions are also introduced by Castellani et al. in [5] where a well known point signature, the *Heat Kernel Signature* (HKS) [10,28], has been extended to describe the entire shape by leading to the so called *Global Heat Kernel Signature* (GHKS). Differently from *Shape-DNA* this approach is based on a point signature that encodes local information. Furthermore the GHKS allows a multiscale analysis that enhances the discriminative properties of the signature. Note that both the approaches [5,26] do not require an explicit registration phase for shape comparison. In [20], a collection of three well known spectral descriptors, the previously cited HKS, the *Wave Kernel Signature* WKS [1] and the *Scale Invariant Heat Kernel Signature* SI-HKS, [3] are computed at every vertex of the mesh and then used in a Bag of features framework for spectral shape analysis of brain structures in order to detect the Alzheimers Disease. The multiscale analysis is instead the basic idea of [32]. This approach encodes the volumetric geometry information starting from the volumetric LBO and obtaining a multiscale volumetric morphology signature which describes the transition probability by random walk between the point pairs and depends on heat transmission time.

Finally, starting again from the LBO eigendecomposition an interesting technique is recently presented by Rabiei et al. in [24]. In this work the *Graph Windowed Fourier*[27] is exploited to encode the geometric properties of the brain cortex. More specifically, a *Gyrification Index* is introduced to represents at every point how much the surface is folded.

Differently from all these methods we propose to move the comparison between shapes from the descriptors spaces to the functional spaces defined on the surfaces. Shifting the focus on functional spaces can be effective and productive as for example in [19]. This work proposes a spectral framework namely *Brain Transfer* to transfer functions between different shapes, in order to explore the shape and functional variability of retinotopy. Conversely, to obtain and analyze this representation we propose the use of the Functional maps framework defined by Ovsjanikov et al. in [22]. This construction is founded on the LBO eigendecomposition and involves diffusion spectral descriptors and their desired properties.

3 Background

In this section we briefly introduce the Functional map framework presented in
[22]. In order to achieve comparison and classification among a family of similar
surfaces it can be useful to recover a point-to-point map T between every pair
X and Y of smooth surfaces embedded in $\mathbb{R}^3$, defined as:

$$T : X \longrightarrow Y, \tag{1}$$

such that for every fixed point $x \in X$, $y = T(x) \in Y$ is the corresponding
point of x. We can consider $\mathcal{F}(X, \mathbb{R})$ and $\mathcal{F}(Y, \mathbb{R})$ the spaces of integrable real
valued functions defined on the surfaces. T naturally induces a map between the
functional spaces, namely the functional map. The functional map for the pair
of surfaces Y, X is a map between their two functional spaces:

$$C : \mathcal{F}(Y, \mathbb{R}) \longrightarrow \mathcal{F}(X, \mathbb{R}). \tag{2}$$

Indeed for every function $f \in \mathcal{F}(Y, \mathbb{R})$ defined on Y the functional map C is
defined by the composition with T as $C(f) = f \circ T$, as reported in the following
commutative diagram:

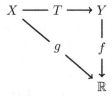

In the discrete setting, given a couple of basis for the functional spaces, C can
be represented as a matrix. Fixing a pair of basis for the functional spaces, as for
example the eigenfunctions of the Laplace Beltrami operator, the functional map
can be represented in this basis reducing the size and the computational cost
of its computation. If T is given than C can be easily computed. Otherwise as
suggested in [22] it is possible to approximate this functional map, adopting a set
of linear constraint optimizations. In our implementation the imposed constraints
are two-fold. The first related to a set of pairs of functions that are stable with
respect to deformations. The second is based on commutativity with pairs of
corresponding operators. In general, the function constraints do not resolve the
symmetry ambiguity, in fact the selected functions are usually symmetric. For
this reason, in addition to the function constraints, in [22] was proposed to add
the commutativity constraint.

$$C = \underset{Q}{\mathrm{argmin}} \sum_{i \in I} ||Q f_i - g_i||_F^2 + \alpha \sum_{j \in J} ||R_j Q - Q S_j||_F^2. \tag{3}$$

where $\{f_i\}_{i \in I}$ is a collection of functions defined on the surface Y, and $\{g_i\}_{i \in I}$ is
the set of corresponding functions to those selected on Y. $\alpha \in [0, 1]$ is a real parameter that allows us to choose how much to give importance to the second constraint. In this way the first part of the optimization function is minimized when

$\forall f \in \mathcal{F}(Y, \mathbb{R})$, that is selected as stable function, $C(f)$ is as equal as possible to $g \in \mathcal{F}(X, \mathbb{R})$ the selected stable function defined on X that matches f. These stable functions can be selected in several way. They can be chosen between the point descriptors that are invariant to isometric deformations. If these functions are known they can be selected as landmark point correspondences or segment correspondences. The second part of the optimization function is called the *Operator Commutativity constraint*. Here for every pair of corresponding operator (S_j, R_j) belonging to $\{S_j\}_{j \in J}$ operators of Y and $\{R_j\}_{j \in J}$ operators of X this minimization force the following diagram to commute $\forall j \in J$:

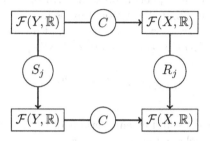

Fixing a proper basis for each functional space, the computation of the functional map can be efficiently done adopting some linear algebraic techniques at the same time also reducing the dimensionality of the problem. For a deeper analysis of the properties and uniqueness of the definition of such functional map refer to [22]. Even though the original method is quite general, in this work we will consider only brain shapes or subparts of brain represented in the discrete setting as a triangle mesh. Concluding this section, we desire to point out that the selection of functions and operators thanks to which we can obtain the functional map is a fundamental step for our work. The choices and the reasons for these choices will be presented in more detail in the next section.

4   Proposed Method

In this section we show the main contributions of our paper that are: (i) the design of a Functional maps framework on the spectral domain for brain comparison, and (ii) the customized Functional maps kernel for brain classification.

4.1   Computing Functional Maps

As mentioned in Sect. 3, we can approximate the Functional map C taking into account two sets of linear constraints. In particular, such constraints are defined by pairs of corresponding functions and by operators that satisfy the commutativity property with respect to C.

In this work we assume that in the absence of disease and disorders the brain surfaces are closer to isometric shapes with respect to the variations caused by the presence of disturbances. Therefore, for shapes belonging to the same class it is possible to find a map T that can be approximated by an isometry. Thus, a good approximation of the Functional maps, in order to detect disorders, can be computed starting from isometry invariant descriptors and operators. This is the motivation that has driven our choices of function and operator constraints.

For the operator commutativity we consider the *Laplace-Beltrami operator* (LBO), a positive semidefinite differential operator, defined on the smooth manifold. The LBO is fully described in terms of the Riemannian metric and therefore it is invariant to isometric deformations of the surface [25]. In the discrete setting the LBO can be computed using the classical cotangent formula [21,23]. As functions constraint we take two spectral point descriptors, which are also selected as probe functions in the original functional maps framework. These descriptors namely HKS and WKS are known to be stable and invariant to isometries.

The first one is the *Heat Kernel Signature* (HKS) [10,28] given by

$$h(x,t) = \sum_{i=1}^{n} e^{-\lambda_i t} \phi_i^2(x) \tag{4}$$

where λ_i, ϕ_i are eigenvalues and eigenfunctions of the LBO eigendecomposition and n is the number of selected eigenfunctions.

In the same way we can define the second descriptor, namely the *Wave Kernel Signature* (WKS) [1], as

$$w(E,x) = \sum_{i=0}^{n} \phi_i(x)^2 f_E(\lambda_i)^2 \tag{5}$$

where E is an approximation of the energy expected value, and f_E^2 is an energy probability distribution.

As extensively argued in [1,10,28] we chose these two spectral signatures because they have a lot of interesting property. The HKS ensures the so called *informative theorem* which states that if X and Y are two compact manifold and the eigenvalues of the respective Laplace-Beltrami operators are not repeated, then the heat HKS is preserved for every isometry T between two manifold X and Y, i.e. $h_X(x,t) = h_Y(T(x),t)$. Although it is possible for some shapes to have some eigenvalues that are very close each others by leading to a switch in the order, in the practical experience the HKS descriptors are quite robust with respect to this non optimal situation.

The WKS is also *intrinsic* and *informative*, i.e. once again for every isometry T between X and Y, we have that $w_X(E,x) = w_Y(E,T(x))$, for every $x \in X$ and for every $E \in \mathbb{R}$ (see Fig. 1). So these descriptors could better represent small variations among near isometric shapes belonging to the same class, allowing a better realization of the functional map.

4.2   Functional Maps Kernel

As shown in Sect. 3, we can estimate the map C for every pair of surfaces (X,Y). For the sake of clarity we denote with $C_{X,Y}$ the map between X and Y. Now,

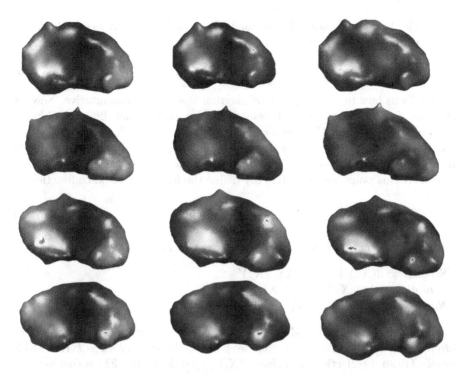

Fig. 1. Distribution of WKS values for several shapes of putamen region and energy values. From left to right $E = 10, 140, 180$. Lines 1 and 2 subjects with bipolar disorder, lines 3 and 4 normal controls.

we need a specific kernel based on this map to perform our classification task. Given the pair (X, Y), we compute two maps: (i) $C_{X,Y}$ defined from $\mathcal{F}(Y, \mathbb{R})$ to $\mathcal{F}(Y, \mathbb{R})$ and, (ii) the inverse $C_{Y,X}$. Clearly the exact Functional map from a functional space $\mathcal{F}(X, \mathbb{R})$ and itself is the identity map Id_X.

If the estimated maps are correct we can draw the following commutative diagram:

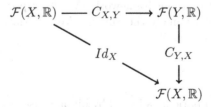

This diagram shows that a function should remain the same when it is moved from shape X to Y, and than put it back to X again.

In order to quantify how well the maps $C_{X,Y}$ and $C_{Y,X}$ have been calculated, we can define the following measure:

$$\|C_{Y,X}C_{X,Y} - Id_X\|_F, \tag{6}$$

which tells us how much the previous diagram is actually commutative. Now we infer that if two surfaces are in the same class, i.e. they do not differ sensibly, we can compute $C_{X,Y}$ and $C_{Y,X}$ in a sufficiently exact way, such that $C_{X,Y}C_{Y,X} \approx Id_X$. Thus for surfaces that belongs to the same class we obtain small value in the Eq. 6, conversely these score will be higher if the surfaces come from different classes. At this point we can advisedly define the following distance function:

$$d(X,Y) = \frac{1}{2}(\|C_{Y,X}C_{X,Y} - Id_X\|_F + \|C_{X,Y}C_{Y,X} - Id_Y\|_F). \tag{7}$$

This distance function has the following nice properties:

- *Symmetry:* $d(X,Y) = d(Y,X)$, $\forall X, Y$.
- *Zero diagonal:* $d(X,X) = 0$, $\forall X$.
- *Nonnegativity:* $d(X,Y) \geq 0$, $\forall X, Y$.

Thanks to this properties and referring to [16] we can define a *distance substitution kernel* on the distance d, that we will call *Functional maps kernel* (FM-kernel). Given a collection of surfaces $\{X_i\}_{i \in I}$ we define the FM-kernel as:

$$K(i,j) = e^{-\gamma d(X_i, X_j)^2}, \forall i, j \in I. \tag{8}$$

As shown in [16] the obtained kernel can be successfully applied in SVM for classification.

5 Results

In this section we show how the Functional maps framework together with our new FM-kernel improve the brain classification performance on the spectral domain. With this aims we explore the comparison with all the spectral methods that are more related to our framework. We also report the results obtained using different classifiers, namely the Support Vector Machines (SVM) and the Nearest Neighbour (NN) classifier.

5.1 Materials

We analyze a dataset of patients affected by bipolar disorder and healthy control subjects. More precisely, 34 control subjects (22 males, 29 ± 5 years old (y.o.)), 34 patients affected by bipolar disorder (15 males, 45 ± 13 y.o.) underwent an MRI session. MRI data were obtained using a Siemens 3.0 T Magnetom Allegra MRI scanner (Siemens Ag). The following parameters were used for T1-weighted images: 256 256 256 voxels, $1 \times 1 \times 1$ mm^3, TR 2060 ms, TE 3.93 ms, flip angle 15°.

Cortical and subcortical surfaces were obtained using FreeSurfer version 4.3.1[1]
[9]. First, non-brain tissues were excluded, then images were segmented into
white and gray matter (WM and GM respectively), and then, meshes of the
boundaries between WM and GM and between GM and CSF were estimated.
We focused on the *putamen*, a deep gray matter brain structure, which is thought
to be modified in the shape in subjects that are affected by bipolar disorder [17].
The process encoded by the functional map framework is shown in Fig. 2. The
function defined on the first shape is represented by the WKS descriptor. Such
function is map to the second shape by using C by showing that the transported
WKS values are very similar to the original one.

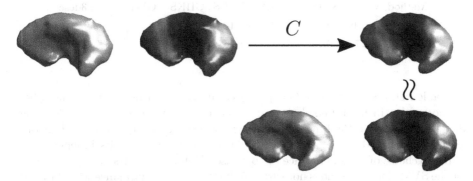

Fig. 2. A couple of putamen surfaces and two WKS descriptors computed on them.
Through the C map calculated using the Functional maps framework, we transport
the function defined on the first shape to the second one and as shown we achieve a
good approximation of the desired function on the second shape.

5.2   Comparison with Other Methods

We compare our method with the state of the art spectral methods. In order to
establish how much the Functional maps framework and the proposed FM-kernel
improve the classification results, we select methods that encode the same information used in our Functional maps construction. We consider the *Shape-DNA*
(S-DNA) descriptor [26], i.e., the increasing ordered sequence of the first LBO
eigenvalues. We evaluate also the so called *Global Heat Kernel Signature* (GHKS)
[5], a multiscale histogram representation of the pointwise HKS. Similarly, we
define the *Global Wave Kernel Signature* (GWKS) based on the WKS. Finally,
since in our method the information coming from LBO, HKS, and WKS is inte-
grated into the same framework we carried out a further evaluation with descriptors obtained by the concatenation of GHKS and GWKS (GHKS + GWKS), or
GHKS, WKS and S-DNA (ALL3desc).

---

[1] http://surfer.nmr.mgh.harvard.edu/.

5.3   Comparison with Different Classifiers

We show the results obtained by different choices of classifiers. Specifically, we adopt a K-Nearest Neighbor (KNN) classifier, with $k = 6$ and the standard SVM classifier using LIBSVM [7]. A cross-validation scheme is introduced to estimate the SVM parameters as suggested in [7].

Table 1. Results in classification for the bipolar disorder on the putamen shapes. The evaluated methods are SVM and KNN classifiers

Classification results						
Method	Ours	S-DNA	GHKS	GWKS	GHKS + GWKS	ALL3desc
SVM	**72.06**	70.59	67.65	69.12	69.12	70.59
KNN	**64.71**	60.29	63.24	61.76	60.29	63.24

Table 1 shows the results. Our proposed approach outperforms all the other methods, also in their joined version. This confirm our claim that performing the classification on the functional space improves the results. Nevertheless, our method performed at best for both SVM and KNN showing its independence from the choice of classifier. Since the proposed FM-kernel is designed specifically for the SVM classifier it does not surprise that the best performance was obtained with this classifier.

6   Conclusion

In this paper the Functional maps approach for brain classification in the spectral domain is proposed. We introduced a specific kernel for SVM classification, namely the FM-kernel, based on the integration among different spectral shape analysis operators and descriptors. We evaluated our new classification method for bipolar disorder detection on the putamen regions by showing very promising results in comparison with other spectral-based approaches. As future works we consider to learn more suitable spectral descriptors for specific tasks as suggested in [8]. In particular, we will focus on the reduction of the importance of the isometry constraint between shapes that is difficult to justify from the clinical point of view even if it is working well in practice. We could also include further information related to the anatomical structure as additional constraints for the Functional maps framework such as the parts of a prior available shape segmentation procedure. Moreover, we will consider that the major variability is for the non-healthy subjects and therefore a new classifier based on the training of a single class (the healthy one) will be considered. Finally, a more exhaustive clinical evaluation will be carried out by exploring other brain regions and by enlarging the cohort of available subjects.

References

1. Aubry, M., Schlickewei, U., Cremers, D.: The wave kernel signature: a quantum mechanical approach to shape analysis. In: Computer Vision Workshops, IEEE International Conference on Computer Vision (ICCV), pp. 1626–1633 (2011)
2. Batmanghelich, K.N., Ye, D.H., Pohl, K.M., Taskar, B., Davatzikos, C.: Disease classification and prediction via semi-supervised dimensionality reduction. In: IEEE International Symposium on Biomedical Imaging: From Nano to Macro, pp. 1086–1090 (2011)
3. Bronstein, M.M., Kokkinos, I.: Scale-invariant heat kernel signatures for non-rigid shape recognition. In: IEEE Conference on Computer Vision and Pattern Recognition (CVPR), pp. 1704–1711 (2010)
4. Castellani, U., Rossato, E., Murino, V., Bellani, M., Rambaldelli, G., Perlini, C., Tomelleri, L., Tansella, M., Brambilla, P.: Classification of schizophrenia using feature-based morphometry. J. Neural Transm. **119**, 395–404 (2012)
5. Castellani, U., Mirtuono, P., Murino, V., Bellani, M., Rambaldelli, G., Tansella, M., Brambilla, P.: A new shape diffusion descriptor for brain classification. In: Fichtinger, G., Martel, A., Peters, T. (eds.) MICCAI 2011. LNCS, vol. 6892, pp. 426–433. Springer, Heidelberg (2011). doi:10.1007/978-3-642-23629-7_52
6. Castellani, U., Perina, A., Murino, V., Bellani, M., Rambaldelli, G., Tansella, M., Brambilla, P.: Brain morphometry by probabilistic latent semantic analysis. In: Jiang, T., Navab, N., Pluim, J.P.W., Viergever, M.A. (eds.) MICCAI 2010. LNCS, vol. 6362, pp. 177–184. Springer, Heidelberg (2010). doi:10.1007/978-3-642-15745-5_22
7. Chang, C.C., Lin, C.J.: LIBSVM: a library for support vector machines. ACM Trans. Intell. Syst. Technol. (TIST) **2**, 27:1–27:27 (2011)
8. Corman, É., Ovsjanikov, M., Chambolle, A.: Supervised descriptor learning for non-rigid shape matching. In: Agapito, L., Bronstein, M.M., Rother, C. (eds.) ECCV 2014. LNCS, vol. 8928, pp. 283–298. Springer, Heidelberg (2015). doi:10.1007/978-3-319-16220-1_20
9. Dale, A.M., Fischl, B., Sereno, M.I.: Cortical surface-based analysis: I. segmentation and surface reconstruction. Neuroimage **9**(2), 179–194 (1999)
10. Gebal, K., Bærentzen, J.A., Anæs, H., Larsen, R.: Shape analysis using the auto diffusion function. Comput. Graph. Forum (CGF) **28**(5), 1405–1413 (2009)
11. Gerig, G., Styner, M., Jones, D., Weinberger, D., Lieberman, J.: Shape analysis of brain ventricles using SPHARM. In: IEEE Workshop on Mathematical Methods in Biomedical Image Analysis (MMBIA), pp. 171–178. IEEE (2001)
12. Gerig, G., Styner, M., Shenton, M.E., Lieberman, J.A.: Shape versus size: improved understanding of the morphology of brain structures. In: Niessen, W.J., Viergever, M.A. (eds.) MICCAI 2001. LNCS, vol. 2208, pp. 24–32. Springer, Heidelberg (2001). doi:10.1007/3-540-45468-3_4
13. Golland, P., Grimson, W.E.L., Kikinis, R.: Statistical shape analysis using fixed topology skeletons: corpus callosum study. In: Kuba, A., Šáamal, M., Todd-Pokropek, A. (eds.) IPMI 1999. LNCS, vol. 1613, pp. 382–387. Springer, Heidelberg (1999). doi:10.1007/3-540-48714-X_33
14. Golland, P., Grimson, W.E.L., Shenton, M.E., Kikinis, R.: Detection and analysis of statistical differences in anatomical shape. Med. Image Anal. **9**(1), 69–86 (2005)
15. Gutman, B., Wang, Y., Morra, J., Toga, A.W., Thompson, P.M.: Disease classification with hippocampal shape invariants. Hippocampus **19**(6), 572 (2009)

16. Haasdonk, B., Bahlmann, C.: Learning with distance substitution kernels. In: Rasmussen, C.E., Bülthoff, H.H., Schölkopf, B., Giese, M.A. (eds.) DAGM 2004. LNCS, vol. 3175, pp. 220–227. Springer, Heidelberg (2004). doi:10.1007/978-3-540-28649-3_27
17. Hwang, J., Lyoo, I.K., Dager, S.R., Friedman, S.D., Oh, J.S., Lee, J.Y., Kim, S.J., Dunner, D.L., Renshaw, P.F.: Basal ganglia shape alterations in bipolar disorder. Am. J. Psychiatry **163**(2), 276–285 (2006)
18. Joshi, S.C., Miller, M.I., Grenander, U.: On the geometry and shape of brain submanifolds. Int. J. Pattern Recogn. Artif. Intell. **11**(08), 1317–1343 (1997)
19. Lombaert, H., Arcaro, M., Ayache, N.: Brain transfer: spectral analysis of cortical surfaces and functional maps. In: Ourselin, S., Alexander, D.C., Westin, C.-F., Cardoso, M.J. (eds.) IPMI 2015. LNCS, vol. 9123, pp. 474–487. Springer, Heidelberg (2015). doi:10.1007/978-3-319-19992-4_37
20. Maicas, G., Muñoz, A.I., Galiano, G., Hamza, A.B., Schiavi, E.: Spectral shape analysis of the hippocampal structure for Alzheimer's disease diagnosis. In: Ortegón Gallego, F., Redondo Neble, M.V., Rodríguez Galván, J.R. (eds.) Trends in Differential Equations and Applications. SSSS, vol. 8, pp. 17–32. Springer, Heidelberg (2016). doi:10.1007/978-3-319-32013-7_2
21. Meyer, M., Desbrun, M., Schröder, P., Barr, A.H.: Discrete differential-geometry operators for triangulated 2-manifolds. In: Hege, H.-C., Polthier, K. (eds.) Visualization & Mathematics III, pp. 35–57. Springer, Heidelberg (2003)
22. Ovsjanikov, M., Ben-Chen, M., Solomon, J., Butscher, A., Guibas, L.: Functional maps: a flexible representation of maps between shapes. ACM Trans. Graph. (TOG) **31**(4), 30:1–30:11 (2012)
23. Pinkall, U., Polthier, K.: Computing discrete minimal surfaces and their conjugates. Exp. Math. **2**(1), 15–36 (1993)
24. Rabiei, H., Richard, F., Roth, M., Anton, J.L., Coulon, O., Lefèvre, J.: The graph windowed Fourier transform: a tool to quantify the gyrification of the cerebral cortex. In: Workshop on Spectral Analysis in Medical Imaging (SAMI) (2015)
25. Reuter, M.: Laplace Spectra for Shape Recognition. Books on Demand, Norderstedt (2005)
26. Reuter, M., Wolter, F.E., Peinecke, N.: Laplace-Beltrami spectra as Shape-DNA of surfaces and solids. Comput. Aided Des. **38**(4), 342–366 (2006)
27. Shuman, D.I., Ricaud, B., Vandergheynst, P.: A windowed graph Fourier transform. In: IEEE Statistical Signal Processing Workshop (SSP), pp. 133–136 (2012)
28. Sun, J., Ovsjanikov, M., Guibas, L.J.: A concise and provably informative multiscale signature based on heat diffusion. Comput. Graph. Forum (CGF) **28**(5), 1383–1392 (2009)
29. Ulas, A., Duin, R.P.W., Castellani, U., Loog, M., Mirtuono, P., Bicego, M., Murino, V., Bellani, M., Cerruti, S., Tansella, M., Brambilla, P.: Dissimilarity-based detection of schizophrenia. Int. J. Imaging Syst. Technol. **21**(2), 179–192 (2011)
30. Vapnik, V.: Statistical Learning Theory. Wiley, New York (1998)
31. Veronese, E., Castellani, U., Peruzzo, D., Bellani, M., Brambilla, P.: Machine learning approaches: from theory to application in schizophrenia. Comput. Math. Methods Med. **2013**, 1–12 (2013)
32. Wang, G., Wang, Y.: Multi-scale heat kernel based volumetric morphology signature. In: Navab, N., Hornegger, J., Wells, W.M., Frangi, A.F. (eds.) MICCAI 2015. LNCS, vol. 9351, pp. 751–759. Springer, Heidelberg (2015). doi:10.1007/978-3-319-24574-4_90

Longitudinal Methods

Volume Representation of Parenchymatous Organs by Volumetric Self-organizing Deformable Model

Shoko Miyauchi[1]([✉]), Ken'ichi Morooka[1], Tokuo Tsuji[2], Yasushi Miyagi[3], Takaichi Fukuda[4], and Ryo Kurazume[1]

[1] Kyushu University, Fukuoka, Japan
miyauchi@irvs.ait.kyushu-u.ac.jp
[2] Kanazawa University, Ishikawa, Japan
[3] Fukuoka Mirai Hospital, Fukuoka, Japan
[4] Kumamoto University, Kumamoto, Japan

Abstract. This paper proposes a new method for describing parenchymatous organs by the set of volumetric primitives with simple shapes. The proposed method is based on our modified Self-organizing Deformable Model (mSDM) which maps an object surface model onto a target surface with no foldovers. By extending mSDM to apply to organ volume models, the proposed method, volumetric SDM (vSDM), finds the one-to-one correspondence between the volume model and its target volume. During the mapping, vSDM preserves geometrical properties of the original model while mapping internal structures of the model onto their corresponding primitives inside of the target volume. Owing to these characteristics, vSDM enables to obtain a new volume representation of organ volume models which simultaneously (1) represents by simple primitives the shapes of the whole organ and its internal structures and (2) describes the relationship among the external surface and internal structures of the organ.

1 Introduction

Human body contains many parenchymatous organs which have internal structures and/or blood vessels within the external surface of the organ. Recent medical imaging devices provide high-resolution volume models of the parenchymatous organs. The volume model of a human organ in our method consists of a set of tetrahedra. The organ volume models are useful for many medical applications including statistical analysis of target organs in individuals and surgical simulators. Here, human organs such as brain surfaces have complicated shape. Moreover, the volume model of the parenchymatous organ consists of a huge number of points. For these reasons, the processes using directly the volume models are time-consuming. Therefore, the description of the organ volume model is important for the medical applications to deal with the organ volume models efficiently.

© Springer International Publishing AG 2016
M. Reuter et al. (Eds.): SeSAMI 2016, LNCS 10126, pp. 39–50, 2016.
DOI: 10.1007/978-3-319-51237-2_4

In the case of the surface models of human organs, one approach for this problem is to represent the organ surface on a common simple surface (referred to as a target surface) such as a plane or a spherical surface by mapping these organs onto the target surface [4,12]. This makes it possible to easily compare among the organs and analyze them via the target surface.

In the case of the organ volume model, in order to understand the structural features of the parenchymatous organ, the model description method needs to represent not only the shapes of the whole organ and its internal structures but also the spatial relations between the external surface and internal structures of the organ. When the conventional mapping methods for the surface model is applied to the volume models, the organ volume is represented as the set of the surface models of the organ and its internal structures. However, this volume model description meets the first requirement, but not the second one.

In this paper, we propose a method for representing the volume model of a human organ with one volumetric primitive with simple shape. The proposed method is based on our modified Self-organizing Deformable Model (mSDM) [6,7]. Unlike the conventional methods for surface model mapping, mSDM enables to map an organ surface model onto its target surface with various shapes while preserving the geometrical properties of the original organ model after the mapping. By extending mSDM, our proposed method, volumetric Self-organizing Deformable Model (vSDM), maps the organ volume model onto its target volume. In the mapping, the surface of the organ is fitted to that of the target volume while each internal structure of the organ is mapped onto its corresponding inner primitive within the target volume. In addition, vSDM mapping preserves geometrical properties of the original volume model such as the angles and volumes of the tetrahedra. The previous vSDM proposed in [8,9] controls the mapping of only one internal structure to its inner primitive whose location is determined manually and fixed during the mapping. Our new vSDM introduces two new techniques: the simultaneous mapping of multi internal structures and the automatic determination of the inner primitive positions based on the structure of each volume model. Owing to these characteristics of the vSDM mapping, the volume model obtained by the vSDM mapping represents the whole organ and its internal structures by their corresponding primitives with simple shapes while describing the spatial relationship between them.

There are several mapping methods for the volume models [3,5]. Li et al. [5] developed a harmonic volumetric mapping for object volume models. The harmonic mapping preserves the length ratio among three edges forming a patch, but not the scale of the patch. vSDM can preserve both the two geometrical properties, that is, the distance along edges between any two vertices. This means that the mapped model by the vSDM describes the spatial relationship among the vertices more faithfully compared with the harmonic volumetric mapping [5]. Therefore, the use of the model obtained by the vSDM mapping enables to find a more reliable correspondence between the volume models. Hu et al. [3] proposed the volume-preserving mapping of a brain volume model onto a spherical volume. The method in [3] controls for moving a few feature vertices in the volume model to their specific locations in the target volume. However, there is no guarantee that the method in [3] controls the mapping locations of many vertices on the surface of the internal structure while our vSDM can map the internal structures with many vertices onto their corresponding inner primitives. From these characteristics, the contribution of our work is that the vSDM can represent a volume model by a simple shape while preserving spatial relations among the internal structures.

2 Modified Self-organizing Deformable Model [6]

In mSDM, a triangular surface model $\mathcal{M}_s$ of a human organ is used as an initial mSDM. For each vertex v in $\mathcal{M}_s$, its 1-ring region R_v consists of the patches p containing v. The closed surface of v is a part of the target surface enclosed by edges not including v in R_v. Moreover, we manually select the vertices from $\mathcal{M}_s$ as feature vertices, and their corresponding points from the target surface.

The overview of mSDM algorithm for mapping $\mathcal{M}_s$ onto the target surface is as follows. The detail of the algorithm can be seen in [6,7].

[m1] Deform the model $\mathcal{M}_s$ to fit to the target surface by the original SDM algorithm [10]. SDM is a deformable model based on competitive learning and energy minimization approaches. Given an organ model as the initial SDM, the model is deformed to fit to its target surface while moving several specific vertices of the model toward their corresponding points on the target surface. The SDM-based mapping is applicable to objects with various shapes as the initial SDM and the target surface although conventional mapping methods use as the target surfaces only a plane or a spherical surface.

Practically, when from the target surface, one point is randomly chosen as a control point, the vertex of $\mathcal{M}_s$ closest to the control point is used as the winner vertex. Here, when the corresponding point of the feature vertex is the control point, the feature vertex is always chosen as the winner vertex. The winner vertex and its neighbor vertices are moved toward the control point. These processes are repeated until all vertices of $\mathcal{M}_s$ are not moved.

[m2] Remove foldovers in the mapped model. This process is derived from the concept in Athanasiadis et al. [1] that if the deformed model $\mathcal{M}_s$ after step.m1 includes the vertices existing out of their closed surfaces, consider that the foldovers on the surface of $\mathcal{M}_s$ occur around the vertices. Based on the concept, we correct the foldovers by repeatedly moving all vertices in $\mathcal{M}_s$ toward the inside of their closed surface:

$$v = \varphi\Big(\frac{\sum_{p\in R_v} A_p g_p}{\sum_{p\in R_v} A_p}\Big), \tag{1}$$

where A_p and g_p are the area and centroid of the patch p. The function $\varphi(v)$ projects the vertex v onto the target surface. If the process is applied only to folded patches, their neighbor patches may become degenerate.

In order to avoid this situation, the process of removing foldovers is applied to all vertices and is repeated until all foldovers are removed.

[m3] If the feature vertices are far from their corresponding points, using Free-Form Deformation (FFD) [11], move each feature vertex to the location of its corresponding point by deforming the region around the feature vertex. When a lattice space is generated around the deformation region, FFD deforms an object with no foldovers by setting properly the lattice for the deformation. Practically, in our experiment, there is no foldover in all the models deformed by our FFD-based movement of the landmarks. Even though the deformed model by FFD includes some foldovers, the foldovers are removed by our foldover removal processing while fixing the landmark positions.

[m4] Deform the model $\mathcal{M}_s$ to preserve the geometrical properties of the original organ surface model after the mapping. In mSDM, We focus on the areas and angles of patches in $\mathcal{M}_s$ as the geometrical features to be preserved. The geometrical feature preserving mapping ϕ is found by minimizing an objective function E_s which is a weighted linear combination of an angle error term $E_{angle}^{(R)}$ and an area error term E_{area}:

$$E_s(\mathcal{M}_s, \phi) = \sum_{v \in \mathcal{M}_s} [(1 - \mu_s)\psi_s E_{angle}^{(R)} + \mu_s E_{area}]; \qquad (2)$$

$$E_{angle}^{(R)}(\boldsymbol{v}, \phi) = \sum_{p \in R_v} \sum_{d=1}^{3} e_{angle}(\theta_p^d, \phi); \qquad (3)$$

$$E_{area}(\boldsymbol{v}, \phi) = \sum_{p \in R_v} e_{area}(p, \phi); \qquad (4)$$

$$e_{angle}(\theta_p^d, \phi) = |\phi(\theta_p^d) - \theta_p^d|; \qquad (5)$$

$$e_{area}(\boldsymbol{v}, \phi) = \left| \frac{\phi(A_p)}{\phi(A_w)} - \frac{A_p}{A_w} \right|, \qquad (6)$$

where ψ_s is a scaling factor to adjust the ranges of the two error terms. θ_p^d and A_p are one angle and area of the patch p included in the 1-ring region R_v of the vertex $\boldsymbol{v}$. $\phi(\theta)$ and $\phi(A)$ are the angle and area of the patch in the mapped model $\phi(\mathcal{M}_s)$. Here, A_w and $\phi(A_w)$ are the whole areas of the original model $\mathcal{M}_s$ and $\phi(\mathcal{M}_s)$.

We decided the four processing in order of decreasing the range of moving the model vertices. In the step.m1, all the vertices are moved dynamically to map the model onto the target surface roughly. The step.m2 is to move all the vertices on the target surface to remove foldovers occurred in the first step. In the step.m3, each landmark is located at its target position by moving only the neighbor vertices of the landmark within the limited space around landmarks. The step.m4 performs the geometrical feature preserving mapping by moving each vertex within its 1-ring region. From the characteristic, our strategy changing the range of moving vertices finds the suitable mapping while avoiding local minimum like Simulated Annealing.

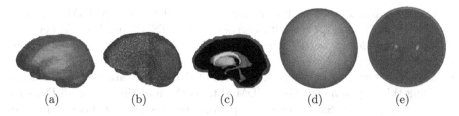

(a)   (b)   (c)   (d)   (e)

Fig. 1. (a) The surface of the brain volume model; (b) The brain volume model cut by two virtual planes for the interior visualization; (c) The brain surface (blue), ventricle (red), caudate nuclei (yellow), putamina (green); (d) The surface of the target volume; (e) The ITS (orange) for the right and left putamina. (Color figure online)

3 Volumetric SDM

In volumetric SDM (vSDM), a tetrahedral volume model $\mathcal{M}_v$ of a human organ is used as an initial vSDM. The external surface of $\mathcal{M}_s$ is regarded as the outer model surface (OMS) of the vSDM. vSDM contains the inner volume models of the internal structures of the organ. Several internal structures to be analyzed are selected and the surfaces of the selected internal structures are used as the inner model surfaces (IMSs) of the vSDM. One example of the initial vSDM is a brain volume model (Fig. 1(a)–(c)) which consists of brain surface (the blue part in Fig. 1(c)), ventricle (the red part), caudate nuclei (the yellow part), putamina (the green part). In this paper, the brain surface is used as the OMS while we selected as the IMSs the surfaces of the right and left putamina.

The vertices in $\mathcal{M}_v$ are classified into three types. OMS and IMS vertices are the vertices on the OMS and IMSs, respectively. The rest vertices are regarded as the inner vertices. For each vertex except the OMS vertices, its 1-ball region is defined by the set of the tetrahedra containing the vertex (Fig. 3(a)).

vSDM is mapped onto a target volume represented by a set of tetrahedra. The external surface of the target volume, called the outer target surface (OTS) is the mapping destination of the OMS. The target volume includes inner targets within the OTS. Each IMS is mapped onto its corresponding inner target surface (ITS). Here, the initial vSDM is completely covered with the OTS. The example of a target volume used in our experiment is a spherical volume model (the light blue region in Fig. 1(d) and (e)) which includes two ellipsoids (the orange regions in Fig. 1(e)). In this case, the OTS and ITSs are, respectively, the spherical surface and the two spheroidal surfaces.

Two main processes comprise our vSDM-based approach to find the volume mapping Φ of the initial vSDM to the target volume (Fig. 2). The first is to map the OMS onto the OTS while moving the inner and IMS vertices to preserve the geometrical properties of the original organ model as far as possible. The geometrical properties to be preserved are the angles of the patches and the volumes of the tetrahedra in $\mathcal{M}_v$. Therefore, the preservation process is called an angle- and/or volume-preserving mapping. The first mapping processes are denoted as ϕ_{mv} in Fig. 2.

The second process is to find a mapping ϕ_m of the mapped IMS by ϕ_{mv} (the green line in Fig. 2) onto its corresponding ITS by mSDM. To perform mSDM, the model to be deformed by mSDM needs to cover the large part of the target surface. Considering this, by using the distribution of the IMS vertices, we determine the position and pose of the LT (the orange line in Fig. 2) satisfying this requirement. The mSDM obtains the mapping ϕ_m of all IMSs to their corresponding ITSs. Moreover, we perform two processes: (1) correcting the inverted tetrahedra in the vSDM and (2) performing a angle- and/or volume-preserving mapping.

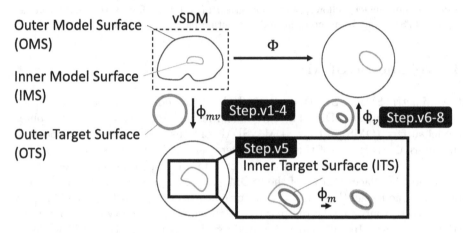

Fig. 2. Overview of vSDM. (Color figure online)

The algorithm of vSDM deformation is as follows.

[v1] Map the OMS vertices of the initial vSDM onto the OTS by step.m1, m2 and m4 of mSDM deformation.

[v2] Move each vertex except the OMS vertices toward the centroid of its poly-hedron. Here, the polyhedron of a vertex v is obtained by removing from its 1-ball region the vertex v and the edges connecting with v. This movement process is repeated until no vertices are moved.

[v3] Correct inverted tetrahedra by **Correction method 1**.

[v4] Perform an angle- and/or volume-preserving mapping by moving the ver-tices except the OMS vertices.

[v5] For each IMS,
   (i) Determine the position and pose of the corresponding LT of the IMS.
   (ii) Map the IMS vertices onto the ITS by step.m1, m2 and m4 of mSDM deformation.

[v6] Move each inner vertex toward the centroid of its polyhedron. This move-ment process is repeated until all inner vertices are not moved.

[v7] Correct inverted tetrahedra by **Correction method 1** and **2**.

[v8] Perform an angle- and/or volume-preserving mapping by moving only the inner vertices while fixing the OMS and IMS vertices.

Step.v1 maps only the OMS vertices onto the OTS while other vertices are distributed within the target volume in step.v2. Step.v3 corrects inverted tetrahedra in the model obtained after these steps. In step.v4, to preserve geometrical features of original model on the target volume, angle- and/or volume-preserving mapping is performed. After the positions of the IMS vertices are determined, in step.v6, the inner vertices are moved based on the positions of the OMS and IMS vertices. Finally, the algorithm performs the correction of the inverted tetrahedra (step.v7) and the angle- and/or volume-preserving mapping (step.v8).

The following describes details of the processes of correcting inverted tetrahedra (step.v3 and v7) and performing an angle- and/or volume-preserving mapping (step.v4 and v8).

3.1   Inverted Tetrahedron Correction

Depending on the shape of the polyhedron of the vertex, the vertex movement in step.v2 and v6 may lead to the self-intersections of the vSDM. As a result, the model obtained after step.v2 and v6 sometimes contains inverted tetrahedra. The inverted tetrahedra provide the wrong description of the spatial relationship among the vertices. In order to obtain the reliable description of the original volume model on the target volume, the volumetric mapping method must guarantee a one-to-one mapping with no inverted tetrahedra between the volume model and the target volume. To achieve this, in the step.v3 and v7, the inverted tetrahedra are corrected by the following two ways.

[Correction method 1]

In our method, an inverted tetrahedron is the tetrahedron whose at least one vertex exists outside the polyhedron of the vertex (Fig. 3(b)). To find the inverted tetrahedron, we use the visibility condition of the vertex from its neighbor vertices: if the vertex v is visible from all vertices of the polyhedron of v, there are no inverted tetrahedra including a vertex v. When we find the vertices not satisfying the condition, the tetrahedra including the vertices are regarded as to be inverted. These inverted tetrahedra are corrected by moving the vertices toward the suitable positions where the vertices meet the condition. To find such position, we check whether the polyhedron of the vertex v is a star-shaped polyhedron or not. When the polyhedron is star-shaped, the polyhedron contains the kernel region in which all points are always visible from the vertices of the polyhedron [2]. Then, the vertex v is moved to the kernel region. Otherwise, when the polyhedron of v is not star-shaped, the vertices forming the polyhedron of v are moved to their kernel region without moving v.

The algorithm for correcting inverted tetrahedra is described as follows. For each vertex v except the OMS vertices, we calculate support planes (the dotted lines in Fig. 3(c)) by extending the faces of the polyhedron of the vertex v. If the support planes form an enclosed region (the red region in Fig. 3(c)), the enclosed region is regarded as the kernel region of the polyhedron. Then, v is moved

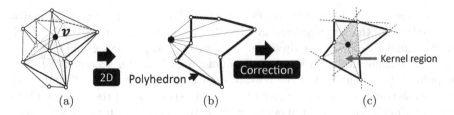

Fig. 3. Example of the inverted tetrahedron correction process shown in two dimensional space: (a) 1-ball region, (b) inverted tetrahedra, (c) normal tetrahedra. (Color figure online)

toward the centroid of the kernel region. Otherwise, the inverted tetrahedra including v are corrected by moving the vertices composing the polyhedron of v to the centroids of their kernel regions. These processes are repeated until all inverted tetrahedra are corrected.

[Correction method 2]

In the step.v7, the **Correction method 1** is applied to the inner vertices to correct the inverted tetrahedra. If after the correction, there reminds inverted tetrahedra in the vSDM, the tetrahedra are corrected by moving the IMS vertices v_l of the inverted tetrahedra along the ITS. To achieve this, by the same way as the **Correction method 1**, we check whether the kernel region of v_l exists or not. If the kernel region exists, we find the quadric surface fitted to the ITS around the kernel region of v_l. When there is the overlapping area between the kernel region and the quadric surface, v_l is moved toward the centroid of the overlapping area. Otherwise, if there is neither the kernel region nor the overlapping area between the kernel region and the quadric surface, we correct the inverted tetrahedron by the **Correction method 1**. These processes of **Correction method 2** are repeated until all inverted tetrahedra are corrected.

3.2   Angle- and/or Volume-Preserving Mapping

In step.v4 and v8, the vSDM is deformed to preserve the angles of the triangle patches of a tetrahedron, and the volume of the tetrahedron. The angle- and/or volume-preserving mapping of the volume model $\mathcal{M}_v$ is to find the mapping ϕ which minimizes an objective function E_v:

$$E_v(\mathcal{M}_v, \phi) = \sum_{v \in \mathcal{M}_v} \left[(1 - \mu_v)\psi_v E_{angle}^{(B)} + \mu_v E_{vol} \right], \tag{7}$$

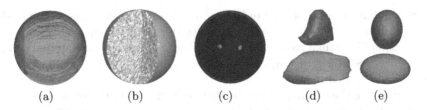

(a)   (b)   (c)   (d)   (e)

Fig. 4. (a) The final model surface with the normals of the original model; (b) The interior of the resulting model; (c) The internal organ mapped on its ITS in the final model; (d) The original left putamen from two different views; (e) The left putamen surface after vSDM deformation from the two different views.

where ψ_v is a scaling factor. The function E_v consists of a weighted linear combination of angle error distortion $E_{angle}^{(B)}$ and volume error distortion E_{vol}:

$$E_{angle}^{(B)}(\boldsymbol{v}, \phi) = \sum_{p \in B_v} \sum_{d=1}^{3} e_{angle}(\theta_p^d, \phi); \tag{8}$$

$$E_{vol}(\boldsymbol{v}, \phi) = \sum_{t \in B_v} e_{vol}(t, \phi); \tag{9}$$

$$e_{vol}(t, \phi) = \left| \frac{\phi(V_t)}{\phi(V_w)} - \frac{V_t}{V_w} \right|, \tag{10}$$

where θ_p^d is one angle of the patch p of the tetrahedron t containing a vertex $\boldsymbol{v}$ in $\mathcal{M}_v$. V_t and $\phi(V_t)$ are the volumes of t in the original model $\mathcal{M}_v$ and the mapped model $\phi(\mathcal{M}_v)$. V_w and $\phi(V_w)$ are the total volume of all tetrahedrons in $\mathcal{M}_v$ and $\phi(\mathcal{M}_v)$. Changing the weighting factor μ_v in Eq. (7) from 0 to 1, the mapping becomes from angle- to volume-preserving mapping.

From Eqs.(7)–(10), the minimization of the objective function E_v in Eq. (7) is replaced as the optimal location problem of the vertices within their polyhedra. A greedy algorithm is employed to find the optimal mapping which minimizes E_v. Practically, one vertex is selected randomly from all the vertices. The selected vertex is moved to a location within its 1-ball region so that E_v after moving the vertex to the location is minimized. The processes of the vertex selection and movement are repeated until all vertices are not moved.

4   Experiment

To verify the applicability of our proposed method, we made the experiment using the volume model of a brain (Fig. 1(a)–(c)). The volume model contains 153,121 vertices and 896,327 tetrahedra. From the internal structures in the brain model (Fig. 1(c)), we selected as the IMSs the right and left putamina, and denote as IMS1 and IMS2. By mapping the brain model onto the target volume with 18,246 points (Fig. 1(d) and (e)), the final mapped brain volume model is obtained in Fig. 4. Figure 4(a) shows the brain surface mapped onto the OTS with the normals of the original model (Fig. 1(a)). Figure 4(b) shows the cross section of the final model in Fig. 4(a). Figure 4(c) shows the internal organs of the final model. Figure 4(d) and (e) show the left putamen model before and after the vSDM deformation.

We evaluate the mapping result by three criteria. First, we count the number of inverted tetrahedra in the final model. As shown in the second column of Table 1, the final mapped brain model has no inverted tetrahedra.

The second evaluation is to verify the mapping accuracy of each IMS, $\mathcal{L}$, in the final model mapped by the mapping Φ onto its ITS, T_l. The accuracy is measured by the distance e_d between $\mathcal{L}$ and T_l:

$$e_d(\mathcal{L}, \Phi) = \frac{1}{2}\Big(\sum_{v_l \in \Omega_l} \frac{H(\Phi(v_l), T_l)}{|\Omega_l|} + \sum_{p_l \in \Omega_t} \frac{H(p_l, \Phi(\mathcal{L}))}{|\Omega_t|} \Big), \tag{11}$$

where Ω_l and Ω_t are the set of the IMS vertices v_l and the points p_l on the ITS, and $|\Omega_l|$ and $|\Omega_t|$ are the numbers of vertices in Ω_l and Ω_t, respectively. The function $H(\Phi(v_l), T_l)$ returns the Euclidean distance between the vertex $\Phi(v_l)$ in the final model and the patch in T_l that is closest to $\Phi(v_l)$. Similarly, the function $H(p_l, \Phi(\mathcal{L}))$ returns the distance between p_l and its closest patch in $\Phi(\mathcal{L})$. The values of e_d for the mapped putamen surfaces are shown in the third and fourth columns of Table 1.

The third evaluation is to verify our angle- and/or volume-preserving mapping by using the angle error distortion e_{angle} in Eq. (5) and the volume error distortion e_{vol} in Eq. (10). In the experiment, the parameter μ_v in Eq. (7) is set to $\mu_v = 0.5$. We define the geometrical preserving ratios r_{angle} and r_{vol} as the percentages of the tetrahedra of which each geometrical error, e_{angle} and e_{vol}, is less than a given threshold. When the average angle and volume of all tetrahedra in the final mapped model are denoted as $\bar{\theta}$ and $\bar{V}$, the thresholds of e_{angle} and e_{vol} in the experiment are set to $0.3\bar{\theta}$ and $0.3\bar{V}$. The values of r_{angle} and r_{vol} before and after Step.v8 are shown in the fifth and sixth columns of Table 1, respectively.

4.1   Discussion

From Fig. 4(a)–(c) and the second column of Table 1, we can confirm that the final mapped brain model has completely the same shape of the target volume with no inverted tetrahedra. Simultaneously, the vSDM maps the right and

Table 1. The number of inverted tetrahedra (IT), e_d of IMS1 and IMS2, r_{angle} and r_{vol} before and after Step.v8.

	IT	e_d of IMS1 $[mm]$	e_d of IMS2 $[mm]$	r_{angle} [%]	r_{vol} [%]
Before step.v8	-	-	-	66.2	63.2
After step.v8	0	3.82×10^{-2}	4.27×10^{-2}	78.1	75.7

left putamina to the elliptic LT1 and LT2 (Fig. 4(d)). The mapped right and left putamina have elliptical shape (the green ellipsoids in Fig. 4(e)), and the differences e_d between the mapped putamina and their ITSs are smaller compared with LT1 and LT2 whose bounding box sizes are $32.6[mm] \times 29.8[mm] \times 53.2[mm]$ and $36.0[mm] \times 29.6[mm] \times 51.1[mm]$, respectively. This result implies that the vertices of each IMS are completely located on its ITS.

Before applying the angle- and volume-preserving mapping in Step.v8 of the vSDM deformation, r_{angle} and r_{vol} are 66.2 and 63.2 [%], respectively. After Step.v8, r_{angle} and r_{vol} increase to 78.1 and 75.7 [%]. This means performing Step.v8 improves the accuracy of preserving the geometrical properties of the original model. As mentioned above, the preservation of the two geometrical properties means that the distance along edges between any two vertices is preserved. Therefore, the final mapped model keeps the spatial relationship between the external surface and internal organs of the original model.

From these resulTS, vSDM can obtain the reliable description of the whole volume and internal structure of an organ with their corresponding simple shapes while describing the relationship among them.

5   Conclusion

In this paper, we proposed the method of representing volume models of parenchymatous organs by their target volumes. The proposed method deforms the OMS of the volume model to fit to the OTS of the target volume while moving the vertices of IMSs within the volume model onto their ITSs. Moreover, we perform two processes: correcting inverted tetrahedra and preserving the geometrical properties of the original model as far as possible. From the experimental resulTS, our method provides the volumetric description of the brain volume model composed of several internal structures which both represents the brain model by the simplified shapes of the brain surface and the internal structures, and describes the relationship among them. Our future works include the verification of the availability of our vSDM by using organ volume models with more complex structures.

Acknowledgment. This work was supported by Grant-in-Aid for JSPS Research Fellow 16J03878 and JSPS KAKENHI 16K00243.

References

1. Athanasiadis, T., Fudos, I., Nikou, C., Stamati, V.: Feature-based 3D morphing based on geometrically constrained sphere mapping optimization. In: Proceedings of 2010 ACM Symposium on Applied Computing, pp. 1258–1265. ACM (2010)
2. Dehne, F.: Algorithms and Data Structures: Third Workshop, Montreal, Canada, 11–13 August 1993, WADS 1993. LNCS, vol. 709. Springer, Heidelberg (1993)
3. Hu, J., Zou, G.J., Hua, J.: Volume-preserving mapping and registration for collective data visualization. IEEE Trans. Vis. Comput. Graph. **20**(12), 2664–2673 (2014)

4. Lam, K.C., Gu, X., Lui, L.M.: Genus-one surface registration via Teichmüller extremal mapping. In: Golland, P., Hata, N., Barillot, C., Hornegger, J., Howe, R. (eds.) MICCAI 2014. LNCS, vol. 8675, pp. 25–32. Springer, Heidelberg (2014). doi:10.1007/978-3-319-10443-0_4

5. Li, X., Xu, H., Wan, S., Yin, Z., Yu, W.: Feature-aligned harmonic volumetric mapping using MFS. Comput. Graph. **34**(3), 242–251 (2010)

6. Miyauchi, S., Morooka, K., Tsuji, T., Miyagi, Y., Fukuda, T., Kurazume, R.: Area- and angle-preserving parameterization for vertebra surface mesh. In: Yao, J., Glocker, B., Klinder, T., Li, S. (eds.) Recent Advances in Computational Methods and Clinical Applications for Spine Imaging. LNCVB, vol. 20, pp. 187–198. Springer, Heidelberg (2015). doi:10.1007/978-3-319-14148-0_16

7. Miyauchi, S., Morooka, K., Miyagi, Y., Fukuda, T., Tsuji, T., Kurazume, R.: Tissue surface model mapping onto arbitrary target surface based on self-organizing deformable model. In: 2013 Fourth International Conference on Emerging Security Technologies (EST), pp. 79–82. IEEE (2013)

8. Miyauchi, S., Morooka, K., Tsuji, T., Miyagi, Y., Fukuda, T., Kurazume, R.: Angle- and volume-preserving mapping based on modified self-organizing deformable model. In: 23rd International Conference on Pattern Recognition (2016)

9. Miyauchi, S., Morooka, K., Tsuji, T., Miyagi, Y., Fukuda, T., Kurazume, R.: A method for mapping tissue volume model onto target volume using volumetric self-organizing deformable model. In: SPIE Medical Imaging, p. 97842Z. International Society for Optics and Photonics (2016)

10. Morooka, K., Nagahashi, H.: Self-organizing deformable model: a new method for fitting mesh model to given object surface. In: Bebis, G., Boyle, R., Koracin, D., Parvin, B. (eds.) ISVC 2005. LNCS, vol. 3804, pp. 151–158. Springer, Heidelberg (2005). doi:10.1007/11595755_19

11. Sederberg, T.W., Parry, S.R.: Free-from deformation of solid geometric models. Proc. ACM SIGGRAPH Comput. Graph. **20**(4), 151–160 (1986)

12. Shi, R., Zeng, W., Su, Z., Damasio, H., Lu, Z., Wang, Y., Yau, S.T., Gu, X.: Hyperbolic harmonic mapping for constrained brain surface registration. In: Proceedings of IEEE Conference on Computer Vision and Pattern Recognition, pp. 2531–2538 (2013)

Reducing Variability in Anatomical Definitions Over Time Using Longitudinal Diffeomorphic Mapping

Daniel J. Tward[1]([✉]), Chelsea S. Sicat[1], Timothy Brown[1], Arnold Bakker[2], and Michael I. Miller[1]

[1] Center for Imaging Science, Johns Hopkins University, Baltimore, MD 21218, USA
{dtward,chelsea,timothy,mim}@cis.jhu.edu
[2] Department of Psychiatry and Behavioural Sciences, Johns Hopkins University, Baltimore, MD 21218, USA
abakker@jhu.edu

Abstract. We address the challenge of variability in the definition of anatomical structures over time in a single subject, using a template-based diffeomorphic mapping algorithm to filter out inconsistencies. Shape changes are parametrized through 2D surfaces, while data attachment is specified through dense 3D images. The mapping uses two geodesic trajectories through diffeomorphism space: template to baseline, and baseline through the timeseries. We apply this algorithm to a study of atrophy in the entorhinal and surrounding cortex in patients with mild cognitive impairment, characterized by rate of change of log-volume. We compare the uncertainty in atrophy rate measured from manual segmentations, to that computed with segmentations filtered using our longitudinal method, and to that computed from FreeSurfer. Our method correlates well with manual (correlation coefficient 0.9881, and results in significantly less variability than manual (p 8.86e-05) and FreeSurfer (p 1.03e-04).

1 Introduction

While post mortem analysis of plaques and tangles in the brain have long been used as the diagnostic criteria for Alzheimer's disease, structural imaging can be important in clinical studies of the disease. The earliest anatomical changes in patients with mild cognitive impairment (MCI) [12] are neuronal cell death in the entorhinal cortex (EC) [7], and have been detected through structural imaging. Atrophy biomarkers measured through neuroimaging have been shown to be predictive of disease onset [24], and are associated with reduced performance on memory related tasks [22] relevant to a patient's lifestyle.

We have been quantifying these early changes through techniques in computational anatomy known as diffeomorphometry. By identifying spatial correspondences between brain atlases and subject scans via smooth diffeomorphic mappings, we can infer information about anatomical changes through properties of theses diffeomorphisms, such as their determinant of Jacobian (see [9] for a recent review).

© Springer International Publishing AG 2016
M. Reuter et al. (Eds.): SeSAMI 2016, LNCS 10126, pp. 51–62, 2016.
DOI: 10.1007/978-3-319-51237-2_5

Estimation of these diffeomorphisms is complicated by high dimensional nuisance variables. The mappings are not uniquely specified in the homogeneous interiors of anatomical structures. Discriminating information is only present on image discontinuities. To address this problem, parsimonious representations have been developed by parametrizing shape changes through a function on the bounding surfaces of anatomical structures, an object of the natural dimension for describing these shapes. In this framework, low dimensional parametric coordinates have been developed by expanding this function in a basis determined through principal component analysis [13,21], or through eigenfunctions of the Laplace-Beltrami operator [20].

On the other hand, the majority of neurimaging data, such as T1 MR images and binary segmentations, is in the form of dense 3D volumes. We have developed a method to incorporate the advantages of the efficient surface representation such as robustness to noise [20] and reproducibility [19], with simple and realistic noise models obtained by working directly with neuroimaging data. These models include white noise (sum of square error) when working with T1 images, or multivariate Bernoulli when working with multiple segmentations [17], as opposed to less easily interpretable data attachment models that work directly with surfaces such as currents or varifolds [1].

Despite these advantages, our ability to infer properties of disease progression is limited by the inconsistency of segmentations of anatomical structures. The problem we address here is the variability in these definitions within a single subject over time in longitudinal studies. This source of variability prevents us from making inferences on an individual level, and mandates larger sample sizes in studies of populations. We address this challenge by extending our framework to map onto each segmentation in the timeseries simultaneously.

This extension has been approached in several different ways. Longitudinal Freesurfer [6,14] addresses this issue with a common initialization of optimization problems for each scan in a timeseries. It avoids modelling any growth or atrophy process with the intention of avoiding bias by privileging a given (e.g. baseline) scan, and to allow the capture of sudden changes.

Several models for growth and atrophy scenarios using flows of diffeomorphisms are discussed in [5], with a focus on modelling populations of timeseries, and describing relationships of a given growth process to a typical one. More complex statistical processes are described through higherarchical geodesic models in [15]. In [11], several parametrizations of these flows are considered, including piecewise geodesic (also used in [5]), spline based, and geodesic shooting (in order of increasing regularity in time).

For our specific problem, filtering out inconsistencies in anatomical definitions, we are less concerned with over regularization and use the shooting approach, using two geodesic trajectories through the space of diffeomorphisms: one from template to baseline, and one from baseline through the timeseries. Such an approach will be shown to significantly reduce this source of variability.

2   Method

2.1   Data

T1 brain MR images from the Alzhimer's Disease Neuroimaging Initiative (ADNI) dataset were examined.[1] Twenty patients were selected, older adults (age 72 ± 8 years), 60% male, education of 17 ± 3 years, with mild cognitive impairment, and having a continuous left collateral sulcus (the most common anatomical variant, others are described for example in [3]). Each subject was scanned up to 5 times, and at least 3 times (so that a residual can be estimated after linear fitting), over 2 years. The EC and immediately lateral cortex (the trans entorhinal cortex, TEC) were analyzed for the presence of atrophy.

Structures were delineated by manual segmentation, on T1 structural scans using the anatomical boundaries described in [8]. The emergence of EC occurs 2 mm caudal to the appearance of the limen insulae and ends 1 mm caudal to the disappearance of the uncus. To account for morphological variation in the limen insulae and uncus, the most rostral boundary of EC was defined 4 mm anterior to the hippocampal head and the most caudal boundary was defined 2 mm posterior to the disappearance of the gyrus intralimbicus, which appears at the caudal end of the uncus. With regard to the medial-lateral boundaries, segmentations were extended as far medially as discernible gray/white matter boundaries would allow and the EC/TEC boundary was delineated vertically at the midpoint of the medial bank of the collateral sulcus. For comparison with state of the art, segmentations were also performed by FreeSurfer version 5.1 that utilizes the 2010 Desikan-Killany atlas [6,14]. We did not use the longitudinal pipeline because the resulting data for the entorhinal cortex was extremely variable and did not look viable.

Imaging data for each subject was rigidly aligned to baseline by minimizing sum of square error in T1 images, and imaging data between subjects was rigidly aligned to a single subject through 4 landmarks placed automatically at the boundaries of the segmentations, minimizing sum of square distances between pairs of landmarks. For each subject i, at time t_j, we denote the rigidly aligned manual segmentation image as J^{ij}.

---

[1] Data used in the preparation of this article were obtained from the Alzheimer's Disease Neuroimaging Initiative (ADNI) database (http://adni.loni.usc.edu). The ADNI was launched in 2003 as a public-private partnership, led by Principal Investigator Michael W. Weiner, MD. The primary goal of ADNI has been to test whether serial magnetic resonance imaging (MRI), positron emission tomography (PET), other biological markers, and clinical and neuropsychological assessment can be combined to measure the progression of mild cognitive impairment (MCI) and early Alzheimer's disease (AD). For up-to-date information, see http://www.adni-info. org.

2.2   Equations of Diffeomorphometry

The background space of an image, $\Omega \subset \mathbb{R}^3$ is deformed by a diffeomorphism $\varphi : \Omega \to \Omega$, which is generated by a flow under a smooth time varying velocity vector field $v : \Omega \to \mathbb{R}^3$

$$\dot{\varphi}_t = v_t(\varphi_t), \qquad \varphi_0 = \text{identity}, \qquad \varphi \doteq \varphi_1. \tag{1}$$

To ensure solutions are diffeomorphisms, the vector fields are modelled as belonging to a Hilbert space of smooth functions V [23], with inner product given by $\langle v, v \rangle_V \doteq \langle Lv, Lv \rangle_{L_2}$ for L a differential operator designed to give smoother functions a smaller norm. Here we implicitly choose L such that the Green's function of L^*L (for * referring to adjoint) is given by the Gaussian kernel $K(x, y) = \exp\left(-\frac{1}{2\sigma^2}|x - y|^2\right)$ for $\sigma = 6$ mm.

This defines geodesics through the space of diffeomorphisms given by Euler's equation. Defining the momentum distribution in the dual V^* as $\mu \doteq L^*Lv$, this can be written as [10]

$$\dot{\mu} = -[Dv]^T \mu \tag{2}$$

We model the family of deformations used to study this population through initial momentum supported on the N_v vertices of a triangulated surface template, q_i for $i \in \{1, \ldots, N_v\}$, that contours our structures of interest

$$\mu_0 = \sum_{i=1}^{N_v} \delta_{q_i} p_i$$

where δ_x is the Dirac distribution centered at x, and p_i is a vector in $\mathbb{R}^3$ parametrizing our deformation. The parameters p will be estimated to model the shape of each structure in a timeseries or population. For notational convenience we write $\exp(p) = \varphi$, for p the parameters, and φ the diffeomorphism calculated by solving (2) and (1). Note that $\|v\|_V^2 \doteq \langle v, v \rangle_V = \sum_{i,j=1}^{N_v} p_i^T K(q_i, q_j) p_j$ which we write as $\|p\|_{V^*}^2$.

These diffeomorphisms act on images through their inverse $\varphi \cdot I \doteq I \circ \varphi^{-1}$, for $I : \Omega \to \mathbb{R}$ an image, which in our discrete implementation is computed through trilinear interpolation. In general we will estimate p by minimizing the sum of square error between segmentation images $\| \exp(p) \cdot I - J \|_{L_2}^2$ for I our template image and J a target image.

2.3   Algorithms

We construct a hypertemplate surface, with vertices q_h, using a restricted delaunay triangulation [2] of the isosurface of the average image of our aligned baseline segmentations. A hypertemplate image I_h is generated by filling each voxel with its fraction inside the surface (estimated by Monte Carlo sampling). We calculate the deformation parameterized by p_h^0, minimizing the cost function

$$\frac{1}{2\sigma_{p_h^0}^2}\|p_h^0\|_{V^*}^2 + \sum_{i=1}^{N_s}\frac{1}{2\sigma_{p_h^i}^2}\|p_h^i\|_{V^*}^2 + \frac{1}{2\sigma_{I_h^i}^2}\|\exp(p_h^i)\cdot\exp(p_h^0)\cdot I_h - J^{i1}\|_{L_2}^2$$

over p_h^0 and the nuisance parameters p_h^i, for J^{i1} the target binary segmentation image of the baseline scan for the i-th out of $N_s = 20$ subjects. The $\sigma_{\cdot}^2$ are scalar parameters that provide the flexibility to change relative weighting between terms, but here they are each set to 1. We denote our resulting template image $I \doteq \exp(p_h^0)\cdot I_h$ and our template vertices $q = \exp(p_h^0)(q_h)$ (i.e. each vertex is transformed directly by the diffeomorphism generated by p_h^0). A diagram of this setup is shown in Fig. 1.

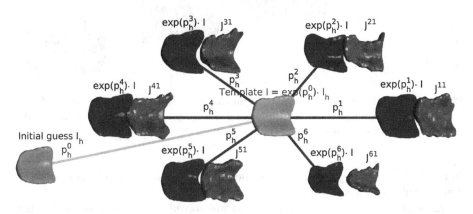

Fig. 1. Illustration of template estimation procedure for six subjects in our population. The hypertemplate is shown in green, the estimated template in cyan, the template deformed to match baseline in blue, and the target baseline scans in red (Color figure online).

Given this template (surface q and image I), we can map onto the timeseries for subject i at each time t_j for $j \in \{1,\ldots,N_{ti}\}$ by minimizing the cost function

$$\frac{1}{2\sigma_{p_0}^2}\|p_0^i\|^2 + \frac{1}{2\sigma_{p_1}^2}\|p_1^i\|_{V^*}^2 (t^{iN_{ti}} - t^{i1})$$

$$+ \sum_{j=1}^{N_{ti}}\frac{1}{2\sigma_{I^j}^2}\|\exp(p_1^i(t^{ij} - t^{i1}))\cdot\exp(p_0^i)\cdot I - J^{ij}\|_{L_2}^2$$

over the parameters p_0^i and p_1^i. The σ^2 again provide relative weighting between terms, and they are set to $\sigma_{p_0}^2 = 2$, $\sigma_{p_1}^2 = \sigma_{I^j}^2 = 1$ (chosen heuristically). For this dataset we express t^{ij} in units of 6 months. A diagram of this setup is shown in Fig. 2, where $I^{ij} \doteq \exp(p_1^i(t_j - t_1))\cdot\exp(p_0^i)\cdot I$. Essentially p_0^i represents the

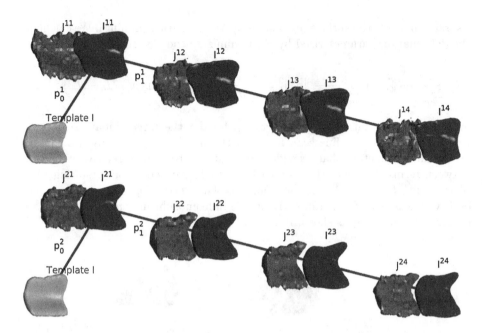

Fig. 2. Example longitudinal mapping results for two subjects. The template is shown in cyan, the deforming template in blue, and the target in red. Top: high variability example, bottom: low variability example (Color figure online).

"intercept" and p_1^i represents the "slope" of a linear regression in the space of diffeomorphisms for subject i.

Each of these minimization problems are solved by gradient descent using an adjoint algorithm. The gradient of each term in the matching cost, namely $(\varphi \cdot I - J)$, is transported backwards in time through a linearized version of the dynamics (1), (2), and $\dot{I}_t = -\nabla I_t v_t$ (optical flow), and contributes additively to the gradient of the the cost function with respect to the parameters. Details of this approach can be found in [20] (or [4] for a similar approach).

2.4 Per Subject Atrophy Rate Estimation

We use the following log-linear model to estimate volumetric atrophy rate in each subject

$$\log v^{ij} = a_0^i + a_1^i t^{ij} + \epsilon^{ij}$$

where v^{ij} is subject i's entorhinal cortex and trans entorhinal cortex volume at time t^{ij}, estimated by summing voxels in the segmentations I^{ij} or J^{ij} (for I, these take value 1 for interior voxels and values between 0 and 1 for boundary voxels) times voxel volume ($0.9375\,\mathrm{mm} \times 1.2\,\mathrm{mm} \times 0.9375\,\mathrm{mm} = 1.0574\,\mathrm{mm}^3$), a_0^i is a nuisance parameter (log volume at $t = 0$), and a_1^i is the atrophy rate (exponential time constant). In this model, ϵ^{ij} is assumed to be independent Gaussian noise with variance σ_i^2.

Each parameter is estimated by maximum likelihood, including σ_i^2 which is the mean square error of the fit. The variance of our atrophy rate estimator is given by

$$\mathrm{Var}[\hat{a}_1^i] = \frac{\hat{\sigma}_i^2}{N_{ti}\sigma_{ti}^2} \tag{3}$$

where N_{ti} is the number of timepoints for subject i, σ_{ti}^2 is the variance in scan times, and $\hat{\sigma}_i^2$ is our estimate of the variance in ϵ^{ij}. Note that (3) agrees with the residual bootstrap variance estimator within 3.3% (root mean square percent error), but in the case that our linear model is incorrect this quantity can still be interpreted simply as a rescaling of square error after the linear fit.

2.5 Evaluation

We evaluate the accuracy of atrophy rate estimates by examining correlation with manual segmentations. We evaluate the variability by comparing the standard deviation (calculated from (3)) of this estimator measured from manual segmentations, to that measured after our filtering procedure, and to that computed from FreeSurfer.

3 Results

3.1 Mapping Results

The estimated entorhinal cortex and trans-entorhinal cortex atlas is shown in cyan in Figs. 1 and 2 (cyan). Two example longitudinal maps are shown in Fig. 2, illustrating a high variability case (top), and a low variability case (bottom). Note the difference in anterior-posterior (left-right on the figure) extent in the manual segmentations (red) for the first two timepoints for the high variability subject. This inconsitency has been filtered out by our mapping procedure (blue).

3.2 Atrophy Rate

For the two subjects shown in Fig. 2, volumetric analysis is shown in Fig. 3. Volumes of the manual segmentations are shown as red dots, while volumes of the deforming template are shown as a blue line. The volume of the deformed template corresponding to each measured timepoint is shown as a blue dot, and the volume of the template itself is shown as a cyan dot on the left. The reduction in variance due to the longitudinal mapping procedure is evident, particularly for the highly variable subject (left).

The atrophy rate estimated for each subject is shown in Fig. 4, with manual segmentations shown in red, the results of our longitudinal mapping procedure shown in blue, and results from Freesurfer shown in green for comparison with state of the art.

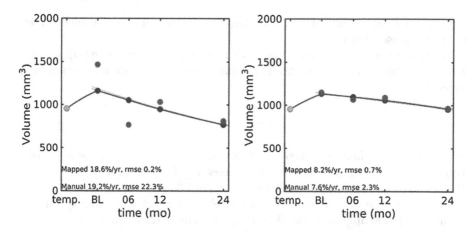

Fig. 3. The mapping procedure's stabilization of volume measurements is illustrated for left: high variability example, and right: low variability example. The horizontal axis indicates months elapsed since baseline scan.

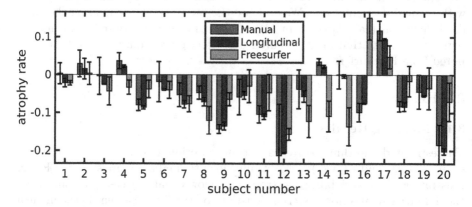

Fig. 4. Estimated atrophy rate in units of exponential time constant, for each of the 20 subjects examined (horizontal axis), is shown for each subject examined as a bar. Standard deviation of the estimator is shown as an errorbar.

3.3 Quality of Atrophy Rate Estimates

Atrophy rate estimators are quite consistent between the manual segmentations and the longitudinal maps (correlation coefficient 0.9881), and not very consistent with FreeSurfer results (correlation coefficient 0.2283), as can be seen in the scatter plot in Fig. 5.

The standard deviation of our atrophy rate estimator, computed according to the square root of (3), is shown in Fig. 6. Significant differences between the three methods are determined by pairwise signed rank tests. Variance is significantly reduced in longitudinal maps relative to manual segmentations ($p = 8.86e\text{-}05$) and relative to FreeSurfer ($p = 1.03e\text{-}04$). However, variance in FreeSurfer estimates is not significantly different from manual segmentations ($p = 6.81e\text{-}01$).

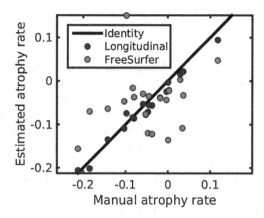

Fig. 5. Correlation between atrophy rate measured from manual segmentations (horizontal axis) and estimated with two methods (vertical axis) in units of exponential time constant is visualized with a scatter plot. Correlation coefficient for longitudinal maps: 0.9881, and for FreeSurfer: 0.2283.

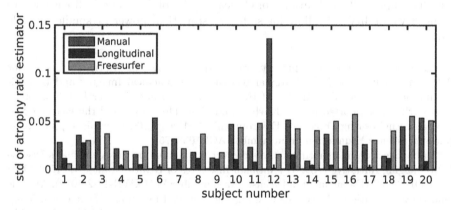

Fig. 6. Standard deviation of our atrophy rate estimator in units of exponential time constant, for each of the 20 subjects examined (horizontal axis), is shown for volume of manual segmentations (red) and volume of our template deformed by the longitudinal mapping procedure (Color figure online).

4   Discussion and Conclusion

As our population of manual segmentations expands to include healthy control subjects in addition to those with MCI, we intend to employ this procedure to identify changes that are specific to disease, as opposed to normal aging. Local modelling of tissue change based on determinant of Jacobian of our mappings will likely prove more sensitive than the volumetry presented here, and can be expanded to include volume change (determinant of 3×3 Jacobian), surface area change (determinant of the 2×2 component of the Jacobian tangent to the template surface), and thickness change (determinant of the 1×1 component of the Jacobian normal to the template surface). An example of early work with this type of analysis can be found at [18].

Because our method treats each segmentation differently depending on its position in the timeseries, unlike the approach in longitudinal FreeSurfer as mentioned in the introduction, the potential for processing bias exists. This was estimated by reversing the order of the timeseries and repeating the experiment, showing an average overestimate in the magnitude of atrophy rate constant of 0.01. This is a small source of error relative to the inconsistencies in anatomical definitions over time we have sought to address. One simple approach for removing this source of bias is to take the average of the forwards and reversed atrophy rates. A second would be to choose the one which produces the smaller value of the cost function. These and other strategies for removing bias will be the subject of future research.

The longitudinal mapping procedure presented here is able to filter segmentation images, significantly reducing uncertainty in atrophy rate measurements, while correlating strongly with raw manual segmentation results. This procedure has important implications for clinical studies of Alzheimer's disease, where reduced variability will allow for sufficient statistical power at smaller sample sizes.

Acknowledgements. This project was supported by the National Center for Research Resources and the National Institute of Biomedical Imaging and Bioengineering of the National Institutes of Health through Grant Number P41 EB015909. This work was supported by the Kavli Foundation. This work used the Extreme Science and Engineering Discovery Environment (XSEDE) [16], which is supported by National Science Foundation grant number ACI-1053575.

Data collection and sharing for this project was funded by the Alzheimer's Disease Neuroimaging Initiative (ADNI) (National Institutes of Health Grant U01 AG024904) and DOD ADNI (Department of Defense award number W81XWH-12-2-0012). ADNI is funded by the National Institute on Aging, the National Institute of Biomedical Imaging and Bioengineering, and through generous contributions from the following: AbbVie, Alzheimer's Association; Alzheimer's Drug Discovery Foundation; Araclon Biotech; BioClinica, Inc.; Biogen; Bristol-Myers Squibb Company; CereSpir, Inc.; Eisai Inc.; Elan Pharmaceuticals, Inc.; Eli Lilly and Company; EuroImmun; F. Hoffmann-La Roche Ltd and its affiliated company Genentech, Inc.; Fujirebio; GE Healthcare; IXICO Ltd.; Janssen Alzheimer Immunotherapy Research & Development, LLC.; Johnson & Johnson Pharmaceutical Research & Development LLC.; Lumosity; Lundbeck; Merck & Co., Inc.; Meso Scale Diagnostics, LLC.; NeuroRx Research; Neurotrack Technologies; Novartis Pharmaceuticals Corporation; Pfizer Inc.; Piramal Imaging; Servier; Takeda Pharmaceutical Company; and Transition Therapeutics. The Canadian Institutes of Health Research is providing funds to support ADNI clinical sites in Canada. Private sector contributions are facilitated by the Foundation for the National Institutes of Health (http://www.fnih.org). The grantee organization is the Northern California Institute for Research and Education, and the study is coordinated by the Alzheimer's Disease Cooperative Study at the University of California, San Diego. ADNI data are disseminated by the Laboratory for Neuro Imaging at the University of Southern California.

References

1. Charon, N., Trouvé, A.: The varifold representation of nonoriented shapes for diffeomorphic registration. SIAM J. Imaging Sci. **6**(4), 2547–2580 (2013)
2. Cheng, S.W., Dey, T.K., Shewchuk, J.: Delaunay Mesh Generation. CRC Press, Boca Raton (2012)
3. Ding, S.L., Van Hoesen, G.W.: Borders, extent, and topography of human perirhinal cortex as revealed using multiple modern neuroanatomical and pathological markers. Hum. Brain Mapp. **31**(9), 1359–1379 (2010)
4. Durrleman, S., Allassonnière, S., Joshi, S.: Sparse adaptive parameterization of variability in image ensembles. Int. J. Comput. Vis. **101**(1), 161–183 (2013). http://dx.doi.org/10.1007/s11263-012-0556-1
5. Durrleman, S., Pennec, X., Trouvé, A., Braga, J., Gerig, G., Ayache, N.: Toward a comprehensive framework for the spatiotemporal statistical analysis of longitudinal shape data. Int. J. Comput. Vis. **103**(1), 22–59 (2013)
6. Fischl, B.: Freesurfer. NeuroImage **62**(2), 774–781 (2012)
7. Gómez-Isla, T., Price, J.L., McKeel Jr., D.W., Morris, J.C., Growdon, J.H., Hyman, B.T.: Profound loss of layer II entorhinal cortex neurons occurs in very mild Alzheimer's disease. J. Neurosci. **16**(14), 4491–4500 (1996)
8. Insausti, R., Juottonen, K., Soininen, H., Insausti, A.M., Partanen, K., Vainio, P., Laakso, M.P., Pitkänen, A.: MR volumetric analysis of the human entorhinal, perirhinal, and temporopolar cortices. Am. J. Neuroradiol. **19**(4), 659–671 (1998)
9. Miller, M.I., Younes, L., Trouve, A.: Diffeomorphometry and geodesic positioning systems for human anatomy. Technol. (Singap. World Sci.) **2**, 36 (2014). http://dx.doi.org/10.1142/S2339547814500010
10. Miller, M.I., Trouvé, A., Younes, L.: Geodesic shooting for computational anatomy. J. Math. Imaging Vis. **24**(2), 209–228 (2006)
11. Miller, M.I., Trouvé, A., Younes, L.: Hamiltonian systems and optimal control in computational anatomy: 100 years since D'arcy Thompson. Annu. Rev. Biomed. Eng. **17**, 447–509 (2015)
12. Petersen, R.C.: Mild cognitive impairment as a diagnostic entity. J. Intern. Med. **256**(3), 183–194 (2004)
13. Qiu, A., Younes, L., Miller, M.: Principal component based diffeomorphic surface mapping. IEEE Trans. Med. Imaging **31**(2), 302–311 (2012)
14. Reuter, M., Schmansky, N.J., Rosas, H.D., Fischl, B.: Within-subject template estimation for unbiased longitudinal image analysis. NeuroImage **61**(4), 1402–1418 (2012)
15. Singh, N., Hinkle, J., Joshi, S., Fletcher, P.T.: Hierarchical geodesic models in diffeomorphisms. Int. J. Comput. Vis. **117**(1), 70–92 (2016)
16. Towns, J., Cockerill, T., Dahan, M., Foster, I., Gaither, K., Grimshaw, A., Hazlewood, V., Lathrop, S., Lifka, D., Peterson, G.D., et al.: XSEDE: accelerating scientific discovery. Comput. Sci. Eng. **16**(5), 62–74 (2014)
17. Tward, D.J., Bakker, A., Gallagher, M., Miller, M.I.: Changes in medial temporal lobe anatomy quantified using probabilistic atlas construction and surface diffeomorphometry. In: Alzheimer's Association International Conference 2015 (2015)
18. Tward, D.J., Sicat, C.C., Brown, T., Miller, E.A., Ratnanather, J.T., Younes, L., Bakker, A., Albert, M., Gallagher, M., Mori, S., Miller, M.I.: Local atrophy of entorhinal and trans-entorhinal cortex in mild cognitive impairment measured via diffeomorphometry. In: Society for Neuroscience 2016 meeting. Abstract Control Number 8556, November 2016

19. Tward, D., Jovicich, J., Soricelli, A., Frisoni, G., Trouvé, A., Younes, L., Miller, M.: Improved reproducibility of neuroanatomical definitions through diffeomorphometry and complexity reduction. In: Wu, G., Zhang, D., Zhou, L. (eds.) MLMI 2014. LNCS, vol. 8679, pp. 223–230. Springer, Heidelberg (2014). doi:10.1007/978-3-319-10581-9_28
20. Tward, D., Miller, M., Trouve, A., Younes, L.: Parametric surface diffeomorphometry for low dimensional embeddings of dense segmentations and imagery. IEEE Trans. Pattern Anal. Mach. Intell. (2016). doi:10.1109/TPAMI.2016.2578317
21. Tward, D.J., Ma, J., Miller, M.I., Younes, L.: Robust diffeomorphic mapping via geodesically controlled active shapes. Int. J. Biomed. Imaging **2013**, 19 p. (2013). Article No. 3
22. Varon, D., Loewenstein, D.A., Potter, E., Greig, M.T., Agron, J., Shen, Q., Zhao, W., Celeste Ramirez, M., Santos, I., Barker, W.: Minimal atrophy of the entorhinal cortex and hippocampus: progression of cognitive impairment. Dement. Geriatr. Cogn. Disord. **31**(4), 276–283 (2011)
23. Younes, L.: Shapes and Diffeomorphisms. Applied Mathematical Sciences, vol. 171. Springer, Heidelberg (2010)
24. Younes, L., Albert, M., Miller, M.I.: The BIOCARD research team: inferring changepoint times of medial temporal lobe morphometric change in preclinical Alzheimer's disease. NeuroImage Clin. **5**, 178–187 (2014). http://dx.doi.org/10.1016/j.nicl.2014.04.009

Spatio-Temporal Shape Analysis of Cross-Sectional Data for Detection of Early Changes in Neurodegenerative Disease

Claire Cury[1,2]($\boxtimes$), Marco Lorenzi[1], David Cash[1,2], Jennifer M. Nicholas[2,3],
Alexandre Routier[4], Jonathan Rohrer[2], Sebastien Ourselin[1,2],
Stanley Durrleman[4], and Marc Modat[1,2]

[1] Translational Imaging Group, Centre for Medical Image Computing,
Medical Physics and Biomedical Engineering Department,
University College London, London NW1 2HE, UK
c.cury@ucl.ac.uk
[2] Dementia Research Centre, Institute of Neurology,
University College London, London WC1N 3BG, UK
[3] Department of Medical Statistics,
London School of Hygiene & Tropical Medicine, London, UK
[4] Inria Aramis project-team Centre Paris-Rocquencourt,
Inserm U 1127, CNRS UMR 7225, Sorbonne Universités,
UPMC Univ Paris 06 UMR S 1127,
Institut du Cerveau et de la Moelle épinière, ICM, 75013 Paris, France

Abstract. The detection of pathological changes in neurodegenerative diseases that occur before clinical onset would be of great value for identifying suitable subjects and assessing drug efficacy in trials aimed at preventing or slowing onset. Using MRI derived volumetric information, researchers have been able to detect significant differences between patients in the presymptomatic phase of neurodegenerative diseases and healthy controls. However, volumetric studies provide only a summary representation of complex morphological changes. Shape analysis has already been successfully applied to model pathological features in neurodegeneration and represents a valuable instrument to model presymptomatic anatomical changes occurring in specific brain regions.

In this study we propose a computational framework to model groupwise spatio-temporal shape differences, and to statistically evaluate the effects of time and pathological components on the modeled variability. The proposed approach leverages the geodesic regression framework based on varifolds, and models the spatio-temporal shape variability via dimensionality reduction of the subject-specific "residual" transformations normalised in a common reference frame through parallel transport. The proposed approach is applied to patients with genetic variants of fronto-temporal dementia, and shows that shape differences in the posterior part of the thalamus can be observed several years before the appearance of clinical symptoms.

Keywords: Shape · Thalamus · Spatio-temporal geodesic regression · FTD · Parallel transport

© Springer International Publishing AG 2016
M. Reuter et al. (Eds.): SeSAMI 2016, LNCS 10126, pp. 63–75, 2016.
DOI: 10.1007/978-3-319-51237-2_6

1   Introduction

The hallmark of neuro-degenerative diseases such as Alzheimer's disease (AD) or frontotemporal dementia (FTD) are the progressive clinical symptoms that include dementia, memory loss, and changes in behaviour. However, there is also evidence of pathological changes occurring much earlier than the onset of these clinical symptoms. This presymptomatic phase of the disease can last more than a decade. Reliably detecting these early changes in presymptomatic individuals could provide the roadmap to improved prevention of these diseases. These findings would not only provide better understanding of the underlying mechanisms of the disease, but they would also result in improved identification of at-risk individuals that would be suitable for potential therapies that will halt or slow down the disease process. Accurate, reliable measurements of these changes could also be used to assess the efficacy of these therapies in secondary prevention clinical trials.

Autosomal dominant forms of dementias provide a reliable means of identifying presymptomatic individuals who are highly likely to develop the disease. The Dominantly Inherited Alzheimer Network (DIAN) and the Genetic FTD Initiative (GENFI) are examples of international studies of autosomal dominant forms of AD and FTD that are collecting multimodal neuroimaging, alongside other biomarkers with the objective of obtaining an improved understanding of the changes that are occuring during the presymptomatic phase of the disease. The structural MRI results from these studies [2,19] have shown evidence of significant volume differences between carriers and non-carriers in numerous regions of the brain years before the expected onset of clinical symptoms.

While the neurodegenerative process has consistently resulted in downstream effects of regional volume, there may be even earlier, more sensitive information, encoded in the shape of the structure. An important aspect of shape analysis is their description. Different ways to describe shape have been proposed. The use of M-Representation [18] allows atrophy measurements and enables the separation of the thickness of a shape from its positioning. However, this representation is sensitive to topological changes. Spherical harmonic decompositions [23] are often used for their simplicity in parametrisation since only a few parameters are required to describe a shape. However, the interpretation of the parameters, and differences between them, is not intuitive. For the current study we represent shapes using varifolds [4], which have the same properties as the current representation [25]. They are robust to varying topologies, do not require point to point correspondences, and embed the shapes in a vector space, which facilitate the interpretation of results.

In this paper the methodology is based on the framework of the Large Deformation Diffeomorphic Metric Mapping (LDDMM) [1,12,24], providing a shape space, there is a continuum between all shapes of the population under study. We develop a for spatio-temporal shape analysis in order to qualify and quantify early shape changes between subjects with and without genetic variants of FTD. We first compute an average spatio-temporal trajectory of the thalamic shapes segmented from a population of 211 individuals [8,11]. Second, we compute the subject-specific "residual" trajectories with respect to the modelled progression, and we subsequently spatio-temporaly normalise them in the baseline reference frame through parallel transport [26]. We finally model the spatio-temporal variability encoded in the "residuals" through kernel PCA. The individual projections in the latent space are statistically analysed via random effect models to investigate significant effects of time and group-wise differences in the encoded longitudinal variability. In the literature we can find different longitudinal shape analysis answering different questions. The work presented in Lorenzi et al. [14] measures brain atrophy for each subject using follow up scans, and the method is not based on the LDDMM framework. In Datar et al. [6] they used a shape representation based on point to point correspondences and tend to model population trend. In Lorenzi et al. [16] they estimate the anatomical age of a new subject regarding to a normal aging longitudinal model based on stationary vector fields. The method aims to estimate from brain images the contribution of aging and pathology. Here the aim of the method is to detect shape differences due to pathology along the time.

2   Method

We indicate with $\{(S_i, t_i)\}_{i \in \{0, N-1\}}$ a set of N shapes associated with a corresponding time point t_i. With analogy to classical random-effect-modelling approaches, we assume that each shape is a random realisation of a common underlying spatio-temporal process $\phi(t)$:

$$S_i = \rho_i(\phi(t_i, B_0)) + \epsilon_i,$$

where B_0 is a common reference frame (typically the baseline image), and ρ_i is a subject-specific "residual" accounting for individual variations, this is the diffeomorphic deformation linking the mesh of the shape S_i to the corresponding time point t_i of the common trajectory. We also assume that ϵ_i is Gaussian random distributed noise. In order to identify group-wise differences between the spatio-temporal trajectory changes, we propose a statistical framework to model and compare the subjects-specific "residuals" ρ_i. This is a challenging problem, since the ρ_i are defined at different time points, and therefore cannot be directly compared in a common anatomical framework. Moreover, the optimisation of the functional for the simultaneous estimation of group-wise trajectory and random effects is not trivial, and would ultimately result in highly expensive numerical schemes. For this reason, we propose to simplify the optimisation problem by introducing an efficient numerical framework composed of three steps illustrated in Fig. 1. (i) First we assume that the "residuals" ρ_i are fixed, and estimate the common trajectory $\phi(t)$. (ii) Second, given the modelled trajectory ϕ, we estimate the random effects ρ_i through non-linear registration between the trajectory point $\phi(B_0, t_i)$ and S_i. (iii) Third, after normalising the random effects in the common baseline reference space B_0, we evaluate group-wise differences and time dependencies. This is achieved through dimensionality reduction and subsequent univariate analysis on the reduced projections.

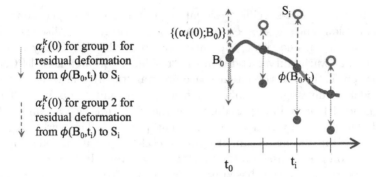

α_i^k(0) for group 1 for
residual deformation
from φ(B_0,t_i) to S_i

α_i^k(0) for group 2 for
residual deformation
from φ(B_0,t_i) to S_i

Fig. 1. Proposed framework. An average continuous shape trajectory is first computed from a population (composed by 2 groups of individuals). Second the "residual" between each shape and the trajectory is computed before being parallel transported to a common time point (B_0) for statistical analysis.

The proposed framework relies on the mathematical setting of the Large Diffeomorphic Deformation Metric Mapping (LDDMM) framework and the varifold representation of shapes. This choice allows a mathematically consistent definition of (i) the spatio-temporal regression, (ii) the ρ_i deformations estimation, and (iii) the normalisation of the initial momentum of ρ_i through parallel transport.

2.1 Large Diffeomorphic Deformation Metric Mapping and Varifold Representation

To quantify differences between shapes, we use diffeomorphic deformations that provide smooth mappings between spaces and are invertible with smooth inverses. The LDDMM framework [1,24] is a mathematical and algorithmic framework based on flows of diffeomorphisms, which allows comparing anatomical shapes as well as performing statistics. The framework used in this paper is in fact a discrete parametrization of the LDDMM framework, as proposed in Durrleman et al. [10], based on a finite set of control points. The control points can be located anywhere not necessarily at the shape vertices, and they are independent of the shapes to be matched. They define a potentially infinite-dimensional basis of the parametrization of the deformation. The vector attached to them define the weights of the decomposition of a given deformations onto this basis, these vectors are called momentum vectors. The position of the control points and the momentum vectors attached to them need to be optimized. The optimisation of the control points concentrate them in the most variable parts of the object to match as shown in Durrleman et al. [7].

Deformation maps $\varphi_v : \mathbb{R}^3 \to \mathbb{R}^3$ are built by integrating time-varying vector fields $(v_t)_{0 \leq t \leq 1}$, such that each $v(\cdot,t)$ belongs to a Reproducing Kernel

Hilbert Space (RKHS) V with kernel K_V, we used a Gaussian kernel:

$$k_V(x, y) = \exp\left(\frac{-|x - y|^2}{\lambda^2}\right) \text{Id, for all points}(x, y),$$

with Id the identity matrix, and λ a scale factor which determines the size of the kernel and therefore the degree of smoothness of the deformations. We define $\varphi_v(x) = \phi_v(x, 1)$ as the diffeomorphism induced by $v(x, t)$ where $\phi_v(x, 1)$ is the unique solution of the differential equation:

$$\frac{d\phi_v}{dt}(x, t) = v(\phi_v(x, t), t), \forall t \in [0, 1] \text{ with } \phi_v(x, 0) = x, \forall x \in \mathbb{R}^3.$$

Velocity fields (v_t) are controlled via an energy functional $\int_0^1 \|v(\cdot, t)\|_V^2 \, dt$, where $\|\cdot\|_V$ is a Hilbert norm defined on vector fields of $\mathbb{R}^3$, which penalises non-regularity. This energy is used as a regularity term in the matching functional. Matching two shapes S and T needs the estimation of an optimal deformation map $\phi : \mathbb{R}^3 \to \mathbb{R}^3$ such that $\phi(S)$ is close to T by optimising a functional

$$E(\phi_v) = d(\varphi_v(S), T)^2 + \gamma \int_0^1 \|v(\cdot, t)\|_V^2 \, dt,$$

where γ balances between the regularity of ϕ and the spatial proximity d, a similarity measure between the varifold representation of $\phi(S)$ and T.

In a discrete setting, the vector fields $v(x, t)$ corresponding to optimal maps are expressed as combinations of spline fields which involve the reproducing kernel K_V of the space V:

$$v(x, t) = \sum_{p=1}^{n} K_V(x, x_p(t))\alpha_p(t),$$

where $x_p(t) = \phi_v(x_p, t)$ are the trajectories of control points x_p, in our case the control points are regularly spaced on a 3D grid containing the mesh of the subject S. The spacing between the control points is defined from the size of the kernel K_V. $\alpha_p(t) \in \mathbb{R}^3$ are time-dependent vectors called momentum vectors. The optimal trajectories between shapes S and T, satisfy the geodesic equations for a given metric on the set of control points such as the varifolds [4]. As a result the full deformation can be encoded by the vector of initial momentum vectors $\boldsymbol{\alpha}(0) = \{\alpha_p(0)\}_{1 \leq p \leq n}$ located at the points $\{x_p\}_{1 \leq p \leq n}$. This allows to analyse the set of deformation maps from a given template to the observed shapes by performing statistics on the initial momentum vectors located on the template shape. The process of generating back any deformation maps from initial conditions $(x_p(0), \alpha_p(0))$, i.e. integrating the geodesic equations, is called geodesic shooting or exponential map and is noted $\exp_{x_p(0)}(\alpha_p(0))$.

As said in the introduction we used the varifolds to represent our shapes [4]. This is the non oriented version of the representation with currents which is very efficient to model a large range of shapes. To represent a shape S as a varifold, the shape space is embedded into a Reproducing Kernel Hilbert Space (RKHS), where it is encoded using a set of non-oriented unit normals attached on each vertices of the shape. As for the current representation, this kernel-based embedding allows to define a proper distance between different embedded shapes. Here the studied shape is the thalamus, which has an ovoid shape, so currents or varifolds could have been used, the orientation of the normals on the shape are not an issue.

2.2   Proposed Framework

The computation of the spatio-temporal regression [8] requires its initialisation to a baseline shape $B_0 = \{x_p\}_{p=1,...,N_{B_0}}$, where N_{B_0} denotes the number of control points defined on the shape B_0. To avoid any bias of the geodesic regression towards an initial subject selected as baseline, we estimate the baseline from the 10 youngest subjects regarding the temporal axis, so subjects with the smallest t_i. The baseline is estimated by computing iteratively the centroid of those subjects in the space of deformations, using the diffeomorphic Iterative Centroid method [5], based on the LDDMM framework.

The spatio-temporal regression of the set of shapes $\{(S_i, t_i)\}_{i \in \{0,N\}}$ is implemented in the Deformetrica[1] software [9,21]. The method requires the discretisation of the temporal axes using T time points, a value specified by the user. The new set of data, used for the regression, is $\{(S_i, t)\}_{i \in \{0,N\}, t \in \{0,T\}}$, where

$$t = \operatorname*{argmin}_{t} \{\|t - t_i\|, \forall t \in \{0, ..., T\}\}.$$

The method computes a geodesic starting at position B_0 at time $t = 0$, and moving to positions $\phi(B_0, t) \forall t \in \{0, T\}$, following the differential equation seen previously, and minimising the discrepancy between the model at time t (i.e. $\phi(B_0, t)$) and the actual observation S_i:

$$E(\phi) = \sum_t d(\phi(B_0, t), S_i)^2 + \gamma \|\|v_0^\phi\|\|_{V^\phi}^2,$$

with v^ϕ the time-varying velocity vector field that belongs to the RKHS V^ϕ determined by the Gaussian Kernel K^ϕ. The initial momentum vector $\alpha(0)$ is defined on the control points of the baseline shape B_0 and fully encodes the geodesic regression.

Then from the spatio temporal trajectory, we compute the "residuals" deformations ρ_i between every observation and the spatio-temporal average shape by estimating the geodesic between $\phi(B_0, t_i)$ and $\{S_i, t_i\}$, using the matching equation seen in Sect. 2.1. We then obtain a set of momenta $\{\phi(B_0, t); \alpha_i(0)\}_{t \in \{0;T\}}$ that encodes the deformations ρ_i from the spatio-temporal regression to all subjects. To make this set of momenta comparable, we need to define them in the same space.

---

[1] http://www.deformetrica.org/.

We transport all momenta into the baseline space of $B_0 = \phi(B_0, 0)$, using a parallel transport method based on Jacobi fields as introduced in [26]. Parallel transporting a vector along a curve (the computed trajectory parametrised by $\{B_0; \alpha(0)\}$ here) consists in translating it across the tangent spaces to the curve by preserving its parallelism, according to a given connection (the Levi-Civita connection in LDDMM). The vector is parallel transported along the curve if the connection is null, for all steps along the curve [15]. We chose to use Jacobi field instead of the Schild's Ladder method [13], to avoid the cumulative errors and the excessive computation time due to the computation of Riemannian Logarithms in the LDDMM framework, required for the Schild's Ladder. Those errors would have been different from a subject to an other, since they all are at different time points of the trajectory, some of them have to travel more than the others. To transport a vector η from a time t to the time $t_0 = 0$, along the geodesic γ, the Jacobian field is defined as:

$$J_{\gamma(t)}(0, -\alpha_i(t), \eta) = \frac{\partial}{\partial \epsilon} \exp_{\gamma(t)}(1/T(-\alpha_i(t) + \epsilon \eta)).$$

The geodesic $\gamma(t)$ is in the direction $-\alpha_i(t)$, and η is an initial momentum vector as the $\{\alpha_i(0)\}$ computed above, is tangent to the geodesic γ at the time point t.

We then have N vectors of size $3 \times N_{B_0}$ defined in B_0. This information is reduced using a Kernel Principal Component Analysis (K-PCA) [22], which is the non-linear version of the standard Principal Component Analysis (PCA). The covariance matrix is defined as:

$$\Gamma_{i,j}^{V^\phi} = (\alpha_i - \overline{\alpha}) K_{V^\phi} (\alpha_j - \overline{\alpha}),$$

where V^n are the eigenvectors of the matrix Γ^V, with K_{V^ϕ} the kernel of the space of deformations used for the computation of the spatio-temporal regression. The n-th mode of variation is defined as

$$m^\alpha = \overline{\alpha} + \sum_i V_i^n (\alpha^i - \overline{\alpha}).$$

3   Data and Experiments

We applied the proposed framework to the GENFI database, using the thalamus as our structure of interest. GENFI is a multi-centre study in which participants come from families known to carry a pathogenic mutation in one of three genes that are the most common cause of genetic FTD: microtubule-associated protein tau (MAPT), progranulin (GRN) and an expansion of the open reading frame 72 in Chromosome 9 (C9orf72). The thalamus is an intriguing candidate for this analysis, as Rohrer $et\ al.$ [19] reported volumetric differences in the thalamus 5 years before expected age at onset. In this paper we used 211 participants, 113 mutation carriers and 98 non-carriers. All participants have a T1-weighted (T1w) MRI and an expected years to symptom onset (EYO). Table 1 shows the demographics of the study participants used in this analysis.

Table 1. Data demographics

	Non-carriers n = 98	Mutation carriers n = 113
Males	59	56
Asymptomatic	98	76
Age in years (med (IQR))	50.2 (36.6–62.1)	52.7 (41.1–62.7)
Years from expected onset:		
≤ -20 *years*	30	21
$-20 \leq$ *years* ≤ -10	16	21
$-10 \leq$ *years* < 0	23	22
$0 \leq$ *years*	29	49

Before running the spatio-temporal regression, we first ran the parcellation of the T1w [3] to extract afterwards the meshes of the structure of interest. Second, we rigidly and affinely aligned the T1w brain images to a groupwise space before rigidly refining the alignment of the thalamus parcellations [17]. Next, we extracted the meshes corresponding to the left thalamus, including around 2, 300 vertices for 441 control points. We have 211 left thalamus meshes associated with the EYO of the subject and the indication if the subject is mutation carrier (MC) or not. For the regression we used 30 time points, which corresponds approximatively to one time point every two years. The space of deformations V was defined using a 11 mm width kernel, which corresponds to half of the length of a thalamus, and a 5 mm width for he space of varifolds.

Similarly to the volumetric analysis performed by Rohrer *et al.* [19], we use a mixed effect model to study the shape difference between the healthy subjects and the MC. The eigenvectors computed from the principal component analysis of the "residual" deformations transported in the baseline shape are used as variables and the fixed effects predictors of interest are mutation carrier status, EYO and interaction between mutation carrier status and EYO. To allow for non-linear change in thalamus volume or shape the model includes a term for EYO^2 and the interaction between mutation carrier status and EYO^2. A random intercept for family allows values of the marker to be correlated between family members.

We did a Wald test on the first principal component, which represents 20.4% of the variability of the residual deformations, another on the second component which represents 11.3% of the variability, and on the third component (10.8% of the variability). We were also interested by the interaction of these components, so we conducted joint Wald test on the two first components (31.7% of the variability), and on the three first components (42.5% of the variability). For each analysis, further Wald tests were conducted every 5 years as in the volumetric analysis [19] to assess how long before the expected onset we could detect evidence for differences between mutation carriers and controls.

The results depend on the metric used for computing the trajectory and for computing the deformations ρ_i. The metric depend on the space of deformation used, which is defined by the kernel K_V used. Choosing a bigger kernel size for the deformation space would lead to different trajectory, with less differences, then to different results. Choosing a smaller kernel size would give a more variable trajectory, leading to different results. The size of the kernel K_V of the space of deformations were chosen to be half of the thalamus size.

4 Results

Results from the analysis of the left thalamus shapes, comparing mutation carriers and controls, including up to 3 principal components are shown in Table 2. To visualise the shape differences between the two groups, we computed two trajectories with the same parameters and the same baseline. One for the mutation carrier group, and one for the control group. Figure 2 shows these trajectories, we can see that the trajectories are indeed similar at the beginning, they progressively differ from each others. At the end of the trajectories, the shapes are clearly different.

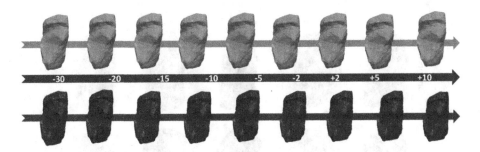

Fig. 2. Geodesic trajectories of the left thalamus, for the control group (first row, green) and for the mutation carrier group (bottom row, red). The figure shows a bottom view of the thalamus. The middle grey line indicates the expected years to onset (EYO) for both trajectories (Color figure online).

Table 2. p-values for differences in the shape of the left thalamus between groups, by expected years to symptom onset and per principal component (PC)

PCs (captured var.) \ EYO	−25	−20	−15	−10	−5	0	+5	+10
PC 1 (20.4%)	0.70	0.94	0.60	0.16	8e-3	<1e-3	<1e-3	<1e-3
PC 2 (11.3%)	0.42	0.26	0.16	0.08	0.03	0.01	0.01	0.03
PC 3 (10.8%)	0.29	0.13	0.08	0.06	0.06	0.08	0.25	0.62
PC 1+2 (31.7%)	0.78	0.80	0.77	0.45	0.07	1e-3	<1e-3	<1e-3
PC 1+2+3 (42.5%)	0.76	0.49	0.23	0.05	2e-3	<1e-3	<1e-3	<1e-3

On Table 2 the first two principal components capture individually significant shape differences 5 years before onset, which is not the case for the third component. The combination of the three components increases the significance of the differences between the two groups and we can then observe significant shape differences 10 years before the expected symptom onset. The results are not corrected for multiple comparison to have a head to head correspondance with the Rohrer et al. [19] volumetric study. We also have strong a-priori expectation that there would be real differences between mutation carriers and no-carriers, furthermore multiple comparison would provide protection against type I error (false positive), while increasing the probability of making type II error (false negative) [20]. Figure 3 shows the first three modes of variation of the deformations, with the information of volume for each component. It can be observed that the first component, which captures approximatively 20% of the variability, does not embed volumetric information. The volume information is however captured by the second and the third component. The first three modes of variation show deformation mainly located in the posterior part of the thalamus, which dorso-posterior part is connected to the limbic system, implicated in frontotemporal dementia.

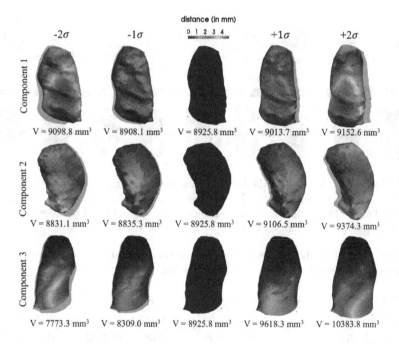

Fig. 3. First three modes of variation captured from the "residuals" between each individual and the average spatio-temporal regression on the whole population. Whereas the second and third components exhibit correlation with the thalamus volume, the first component exhibits a constant volume. It can be observed that the captured variations is located in the posterior part of the thalamus.

5 Conclusion

Using the proposed framework for spatio-temporal shape analysis, we have been able to detect shape differences 10 years before the expected onset of clinical symptoms associated with frontotemporal dementia. Using volumetric information alone, Rohrer *et al.* [19] were able to detect statistical differences 5 years prior to clinical onset using the same statistical analysis method. Not only does the proposed framework provide the potential for more sensitivity, but it also allows for better spatial localisation of the changes within the structure. As shown by the first mode of variation captured from the data, there are differences between the groups that are not captured by the volumetric information. These differences are located in the posterior part of the thalamus. In this study, we focused on the left thalamus. In the future we will investigate how much information can be extracted from other regions of interest that exhibited volumetric differences. We will also further enhance our framework to include longitudinal information with the aim to better capture the shape differences between the groups.

Acknowledgements. Claire Cury is supported by the EU-FP7 project VPH-DARE@IT (FP7-ICT-2011-9-601055). Marco Lorenzi received funding from the EPSRC (EP/J020990/1). Jennifer Nicholas is supported by UK Medical Research Council (grant MR/M023664/1). David Cash is supported by grants from the Alzheimer Society (AS-PG-15-025), Alzheimers Research UK (ARUK-PG2014-1946) and Medical Research Council UK (MR/M023664/1). Stanley Durrleman has received funding from the program Investissements d'avenir ANR-10-IAIHU-06 and the European Unions Horizon 2020 research and innovation programme EuroPOND under grant agreement No. 666992. Jonathan D. Rohrer is an MRC Clinician Scientist and has received funding from the NIHR Rare Diseases Translational Research Collaboration. Sebastien Ourselin receives funding from the EPSRC (EP/H046410/1, EP/K005278), the MRC (MR/J01107X/1), the NIHR Biomedical Research Unit (Dementia) at UCL and the National Institute for Health Research University College London Hospitals Biomedical Research Centre (NIHR BRC UCLH/UCL High Impact Initiative-BW.mn.BRC10269). Marc Modat is supported by the UCL Leonard Wolfson Experimental Neurology Centre (PR/ylr/18575) and Alzheimers Society UK (AS-PG-15-025). We would like to thank the participants and their families for taking part in the GENFI study.

References

1. Beg, M.F., Miller, M.I., Trouvé, A., Younes, L.: Computing large deformation metric mappings via geodesic flows of diffeomorphisms. Int. J. Comput. Vis. **61**(2), 139–157 (2005)
2. Benzinger, T.L.S., Blazey, T., Jack, C.R., et al.: Regional variability of imaging biomarkers in autosomal dominant Alzheimer's disease. Proc. Natl. Acad. Sci. **110**(47), E4502–E4509 (2013)

3. Cardoso, M.J., Leung, K., Modat, M., Keihaninejad, S., Cash, D., Barnes, J., Fox, N.C., Ourselin, S., ADNI: STEPS: similarity and truth estimation for propagated segmentations and its application to hippocampal segmentation and brain parcelation. Med. Image Anal. **17**(6), 671–684 (2013)
4. Charon, N., Trouvé, A.: The varifold representation of nonoriented shapes for diffeomorphic registration. SIAM J. Imaging Sci. **6**(4), 2547–2580 (2013)
5. Cury, C., Glaunès, J.A., Colliot, O.: Diffeomorphic iterative centroid methods for template estimation on large datasets. In: Nielsen, F. (ed.) Geometric Theory of Information. Signals and Communication Technology, pp. 273–299. Springer International Publishing, Heidelberg (2014)
6. Datar, M., Muralidharan, P., Kumar, A., Gouttard, S., Piven, J., Gerig, G., Whitaker, R., Fletcher, P.T.: Mixed-effects shape models for estimating longitudinal changes in anatomy. In: Durrleman, S., Fletcher, T., Gerig, G., Niethammer, M. (eds.) STIA 2012. LNCS, vol. 7570, pp. 76–87. Springer, Heidelberg (2012). doi:10.1007/978-3-642-33555-6_7
7. Durrleman, S., Allassonnire, S., Joshi, S.: Sparse adaptive parameterization of variability in image ensembles. Int. J. Comput. Vis. **101**(1), 161–183 (2013)
8. Durrleman, S., Pennec, X., Trouvé, A., Braga, J., Gerig, G., Ayache, N.: Toward a comprehensive framework for the spatiotemporal statistical analysis of longitudinal shape datas. Int. J. Comput. Vis. **103**(1), 22–59 (2013)
9. Durrleman, S., Prastawa, M., Charon, N., Korenberg, J.R., Joshi, S., Gerig, G., Trouvé, A.: Morphometry of anatomical shape complexes with dense deformations and sparse parameters. NeuroImage **101**, 35–49 (2014)
10. Durrleman, S., Prastawa, M., Gerig, G., Joshi, S.: Optimal data-driven sparse parameterization of diffeomorphisms for population analysis. In: Székely, G., Hahn, H.K. (eds.) IPMI 2011. LNCS, vol. 6801, pp. 123–134. Springer, Heidelberg (2011). doi:10.1007/978-3-642-22092-0_11
11. Fishbaugh, J., Prastawa, M., Gerig, G., Durrleman, S.: Geodesic shape regression in the framework of currents. In: Gee, J.C., Joshi, S., Pohl, K.M., Wells, W.M., Zöllei, L. (eds.) IPMI 2013. LNCS, vol. 7917, pp. 718–729. Springer, Heidelberg (2013). doi:10.1007/978-3-642-38868-2_60
12. Glaunès, J., Qiu, A., Miller, M.I., Younes, L.: Large deformation diffeomorphic metric curve mapping. Int. J. Comput. Vis. **80**(3), 317–336 (2008)
13. Kheyfets, A., Miller, W.A., Newton, G.A.: Schild's ladder parallel transport procedure for an arbitrary connection. Int. J. Theor. Phys. **39**(12), 2891–2898 (2000)
14. Lorenzi, M., Ayache, N., Frisoni, G., Pennec, X., et al.: 4D registration of serial brain's MR images: a robust measure of changes applied to Alzheimer's disease. In: MICCAI Workshop, Challenge on Computer-Aided Diagnosis of Dementia Based on Structural MRI Data (2010)
15. Lorenzi, M., Pennec, X.: Efficient parallel transport of deformations in time series of images: from schilds to pole ladder. J. Math. Imaging Vis. **50**(1–2), 5–17 (2013)
16. Lorenzi, M., Pennec, X., Frisoni, G.B., Ayache, N.: Disentangling normal aging from Alzheimer's disease in structural magnetic resonance images. Neurobiol. Aging **36**, S42–S52 (2015)
17. Modat, M., Cash, D.M., Daga, P., Winston, G.P., Duncan, J.S., Ourselin, S.: Global image registration using a symmetric block-matching approach. J. Med. Imaging **1**(2), 024003–024003 (2014)
18. Pizer, S.M., Fletcher, P.T., Joshi, S., Thall, A., Chen, J.Z., Fridman, Y., Fritsch, D.S., Gash, A.G., Glotzer, J.M., Jiroutek, M.R., Lu, C., Muller, K.E., Tracton, G., Yushkevich, P., Chaney, E.L.: Deformable M-reps for 3D medical image segmentations. Int. J. Comput. Vis. **55**(2–3), 85–106 (2003)

19. Rohrer, J.D., Nicholas, J.M., Cash, D.M., van Swieten, J., Dopper, E., Jiskoot, L., van Minkelen, R., Serge A Rombouts, M.J.C., Clegg, S., Espak, M., Mead, S., Thomas, D.L., Vita, E.D., et al.: Presymptomatic cognitive and neuroanatomical changes in genetic frontotemporal dementia in the Genetic Frontotemporal dementia Initiative (GENFI) study: a cross-sectional analysis. Lancet Neurol. **14**(3), 253–262 (2015)
20. Rothman, K.J.: No adjustments are needed for multiple comparisons. Epidemiology (Cambridge, Mass.) **1**(1), 43–46 (1990)
21. Routier, A., Gori, P., Fouquier, A.B.G., Lecomte, S., Colliot, O., Durrleman, S.: Evaluation of morphometric descriptors of deep brain structures for the automatic classification of patients with Alzheimer's disease, mild cognitive impairment and elderly controls. In: MICCAI Workshop, Challenge on Computer-Aided Diagnosis of Dementia Based on Structural MRI Data, September 2014
22. Schölkopf, B., Smola, A., Müller, K.R.: Nonlinear component analysis as a kernel eigenvalue problem. Neural Comput. **10**(5), 1299–1319 (1998)
23. Styner, M., Oguz, I., Xu, S., Brechbühler, C., Pantazis, D., Levitt, J.J., Shenton, M.E., Gerig, G.: Framework for the statistical shape analysis of brain structures using SPHARM-PDM. Insight J. **1071**, 242–250 (2006)
24. Trouvé, A.: Diffeomorphisms groups and pattern matching in image analysis. Int. J. Comput. Vis. **28**(3), 213–221 (1998)
25. Vaillant, M., Glaunès, J.: Surface matching via currents. In: Christensen, G.E., Sonka, M. (eds.) IPMI 2005. LNCS, vol. 3565, pp. 381–392. Springer, Heidelberg (2005). doi:10.1007/11505730_32
26. Younes, L.: Jacobi fields in groups of diffeomorphisms and applications. Q. Appl. Math. **65**, 113–134 (2007)

Shape Methods

Longitudinal Scoliotic Trunk Analysis via Spectral Representation and Statistical Analysis

Ola Ahmad[1,2](✉), Herve Lombaert[3], Stefan Parent[1,2], Hubert Labelle[1,2],
Jean Dansereau[2,4], and Farida Cheriet[2,4]

[1] Université de Montréal, Montréal, Canada
olasahmad@gmail.com
[2] Centre de Recherche du CHU Sainte-Justine, Montréal, Canada
[3] INRIA, Sophia-antipolis, France
[4] École Polytechnique de Montréal, Montréal, Canada

Abstract. Scoliosis is a complex 3D deformation of the spine leading to asymmetry of the external shape of the human trunk. A clinical follow-up of this deformation is decisive for its treatment, which depends on the spinal curvature but also on the deformity's progression over time. This paper presents a new method for longitudinal analysis of scoliotic trunks based on spectral representation of shapes combined with statistical analysis. The spectrum of the surface model is used to compute the correspondence between deformable scoliotic trunks. Spectral correspondence is combined with Canonical Correlation Analysis to do point-wise feature comparison between models. This novel combination allows us to efficiently capture within-subject shape changes to assess scoliosis progression (SP). We tested our method on 23 scoliotic patients with right thoracic curvature. Quantitative comparison with spinal measurements confirms that our method is able to identify significant changes associated with SP.

1   Introduction

Scoliosis is a complex 3D deformation affecting the general appearance of torso shape. This deformation is defined by abnormal curvature of the spine accompanied by deformation of the rib cage. The standard evaluation protocols of this pathology use clinical measurements such as the Cobb Angle (CA) [7], which is based on radiographic image data and quantifies the severity of the spinal curvature. Scoliosis is more commonly diagnosed in children aged 10–18 years and may develop rapidly, to the point of requiring surgical intervention. Frequent observations are therefore required to monitor the condition during the adolescent growth spurt. An increase in CA of more than 6° indicates a worsening of the curvature [21]. But since the CA is limited to spinal curvature assessment, this measure cannot evaluate the complex deformation of the torso shape. Yet, the importance of the latter should not be underestimated as it exhibits the first symptoms of scoliosis and is the major concern for adolescent patients. Scoliosis manifests itself in shape asymmetries and a high variety of deformations of the

M. Reuter et al. (Eds.): SeSAMI 2016, LNCS 10126, pp. 79–91, 2016.
DOI: 10.1007/978-3-319-51237-2_7

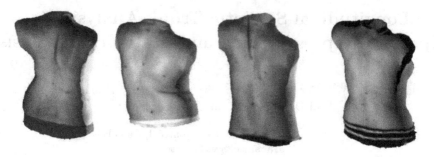

Fig. 1. Sample scoliotic trunk surfaces of different patients. These examples illustrate the high variability in the shape of scoliotic trunks.

external surface of the trunk. These anomalies include deformations such as a hump at the back, a lateral shift of the trunk and asymmetries of the shoulders, scapulae, waist and hips (Fig. 1). Analysis of the scoliotic trunk shape is valuable in the clinical setting to assess the effect of surgical correction or to monitor scoliosis progression (SP), i.e. the worsening of the deformation over time. A clinical follow-up of scoliotic 3D shape deformities therefore becomes decisive for its management.

Previous approaches based on cross-sectional trunk surface analysis either describe back rotation and lateral shifts of the trunk [18,22], or quantify torso shape by three rotations in the lateral, axial and posterior-anterior planes [3]. They ignore all the local deformations of scoliotic shapes, and consequently, are limited in detecting SP. Statistical shape models [1] have been recently proposed to evaluate local shape deformations of scoliotic trunks. These models are trained on populations of normal shapes in a reduced feature space. However, the reduced space affects the statistical power of these models to reveal SP. Furthermore, these models are often biased by the control groups used to train them, and may not account for large shape variations due to normal variability across a population and to anatomical growth, as is the case in adolescents.

To overcome these issues, we propose a longitudinal analysis of scoliotic trunks based on spectral representation and statistical analysis of shapes. More specifically, a statistical shape analysis will incorporate within-subject spectral correspondence of surface models. Currently, spectral methods provide efficient tools for the representation of geometric models, e.g., meshes, shape matching [8,12,13,20], segmentation [19] and registration [15,19]. Shape spectra are isometry-invariant and are more robust to large deformations of surface models. They are considered as fingerprints of shapes [20]. Accordingly, matching shapes in the spectral domain enables accurate correspondence independently from their spatial positions in the Euclidean space. We exploit the spectral matching framework to compute correspondence between scoliotic trunk surfaces. A robust correspondence facilitates the underlying statistical analysis problem, in particular, detecting local changes between shapes. Change detection approaches in longitudinal processing provide numerous statistical tools to capture significant differences, for instance, associated with disease progression [9] and pattern evolution [2]. Inspired by these methods, we propose the Canonical Correlation Analysis (CCA) method [11] to evaluate point-wise differences between matched shapes. Performing this analysis within subjects is useful to assess SP during clinical follow-up protocols.

We begin this paper by describing the representation of scoliotic trunks via the spectral graph. To our knowledge, this is the first time that the spectrum of the graph is used for scoliotic trunk analysis. We exploit the recent work on spectral matching [14] to find accurate correspondence maps between shape models. Spectral correspondence, together with CCA, are proposed for efficient point-wise feature comparison between longitudinally acquired scoliotic trunk shapes. We tested our method using the clinical follow-up trunk shape data of a set of patients with a specific type of scoliotic curvature: right thoracic spinal curve. Our results, when validated versus standard clinical measurements, show that significant shape changes revealed by this novel method of analysis are associated with SP.

2   Method

2.1   Spectral Representation of Trunk Surfaces

Let us assume a discrete representation of the trunk surface as a triangulated mesh. A spectral representation of the surface is then derived using the general Laplacian operator on a graph. Let $\mathcal{G} = \{\mathcal{V}, \mathcal{E}\}$ be a graph defined by the set of vertices, with spatial coordinates $\mathbf{x} = (x, y, z)^T$, and the set of edges connecting pairs of neighboring vertices. The general graph Laplacian is then formulated as $\mathcal{L} = G^{-1}(D - W)$, where W is the $|\mathcal{V}| \times |\mathcal{V}|$ weighted adjacency matrix, D is the diagonal degree matrix defined as $D_{ii} = \sum_j W_{ij}$, and G is the diagonal matrix of vertex weights, defined as $G = D$. Our weighted adjacency matrix is defined by the heat kernel $W_{ij} = \exp^{-\|\mathbf{x}_i - \mathbf{x}_j\|^2 / 2\sigma^2}$ ($\sigma \in \mathbb{R}$), if there is an edge connecting vertices i and j, i.e., $e_{ij} \in \mathcal{E}$; otherwise $W_{ij} = 0$. The harmonic spectrum of the shape of scoliotic trunks (see Fig. 2) is obtained from the generalized eigenvector problem $\mathcal{L} = \mathbf{U}\Lambda\mathbf{U}^{-1}$, where $\Lambda = \operatorname{diag}(\lambda_0, \lambda_1, ..., \lambda_{|\mathcal{V}|})$ are the ordered eigenvalues and $\mathbf{U} = (U_0, U_1, ..., U_{|\mathcal{V}|})$ are their associated eigenfunctions. If the graph is connected, the first eigenvalue λ_0 is always equal to zero [4], i.e. there is no boundary condition, and the first eigenfunction U_0 is always constant. This solution is valid for trunk surfaces, since meshes are interpolated[1] to fill the holes where the trunk model is cropped off, i.e. at the arms, neck and pelvis. We leave out the first (trivial) eigenfunction corresponding to the zero eigenvalue, so that $\mathbf{U} = (U_1, ..., U_{|\mathcal{V}|})$ and λ_1 becomes the first non-zero eigenvalue of Λ. Accordingly, each mesh vertex $\mathbf{x}$ is represented in the spectral domain by the embedding $(\lambda_1^{-1/2}U_1(\mathbf{x}), ..., \lambda_K^{-1/2}U_K(\mathbf{x}))$—a row of the matrix $\mathbf{U}\Lambda^{-1/2}$.

---

[1] The Radial Basis Functions (RBF) algorithm [6] is used to interpolate incomplete trunk meshes and to enforce mesh connectivity.

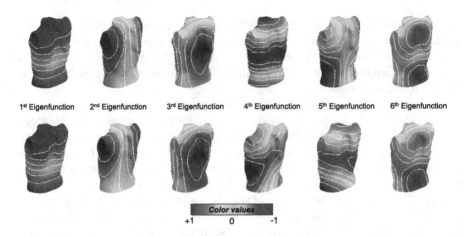

Fig. 2. Spectral representation: the first 6 eigenfunctions of the trunk shape of a patient at two different times. Eigenfunctions 2–6 are incompatible between surfaces due to sign flips and changes in the eigenfunctions. Direct matching between surfaces will thus be inconsistent. White isolines highlight the instabilities between eigenfunctions. The color scale indicates harmonic (eigenfunction) amplitude in the spectral domain. (Color figure online)

2.2   Spectral Correspondence Between Trunk Surfaces

The spectral representation defines a feature space to solve the correspondence problem between shapes via spectral matching. Spectral correspondence must however ensure stability between matched shapes [13]. Figure 2 shows incompatibility in harmonic bases 2–6 between surface models, manifested by sign flips as well as changes in the shape and orientation of the eigenfunctions, due to numerical instabilities and multiplicity ambiguities in the eigenvalues. In more recent work [14], the correspondence problem has been addressed efficiently by the transfer of harmonic weights $\Lambda^{-1/2}$ across shapes. We apply this method to find the correspondence between pairs of scoliotic trunk shapes. Let two meshes M_1 and M_2 represent the surface models of a deformable scoliotic trunk. (The term "deformable" here refers to the fact that a patient's trunk shape changes over time.) Their spectral representations can thus be defined as $\mathbf{U}_1 \Lambda_1^{-1/2}$ and $\mathbf{U}_2 \Lambda_2^{-1/2}$, respectively. The spectral transfer from M_1 to M_2 is defined by the $K \times K$ matrix

$$R_{12} = \left((\mathbf{U}_2)^T \mathbf{U}_2\right)^{-1} \left((\mathbf{U}_2)^T \mathbf{U}_{(1 \circ c)}\right) \tag{1}$$

where c is the unknown correspondence map such that $\mathbf{U}_{(1 \circ c)} \Lambda_1^{-1/2}$ is equivalent to $\mathbf{U}_2 R_{12} \Lambda_2^{-1/2}$. The correspondence c is solved as an optimization problem (detailed in [14]) that minimizes the l_2 norm of the difference

$$c = \mathrm{argmin}_c \| \mathbf{U}_{(1 \circ c)} \Lambda_1^{-1/2} - \mathbf{U}_2 R_{12} \Lambda_2^{-1/2} \|^2. \tag{2}$$

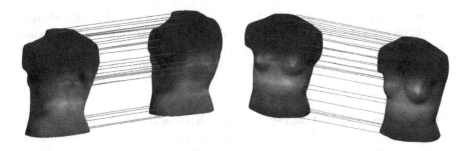

Fig. 3. Spectral correspondence resulting from the transfer of harmonic weights between two scoliotic trunks. Similar colors represent corresponding points in the posterior (left) and anterior (right) views of the trunk surfaces. Regions of the deformable shapes exhibiting local variability, e.g. the shoulders, scapulae, hips and waist, are correctly matched. (Color figure online)

Similarly, the inverse correspondence c^{-1} that maps mesh M_2 to mesh M_1 can be solved such that $\mathbf{U}_{(2\circ c^{-1})}\Lambda_2^{-1/2}$ is equivalent to $\mathbf{U}_1 R_{21}\Lambda_1^{-1/2}$, where

$$R_{21} = \left((\mathbf{U}_1)^T \mathbf{U}_1\right)^{-1}\left((\mathbf{U}_1)^T \mathbf{U}_{(2\circ c^{-1})}\right) \tag{3}$$

is the $K \times K$ spectral transfer matrix from M_2 to M_1. To enforce symmetry in the solution, both c and c^{-1} are used in the underlying energy function. The number of harmonic bases K determines the resolution used to compute the correspondence in the spectral domain. Since trunk shapes are smooth surfaces, it was sufficient in our experiments to compute the correspondence between their meshes using at most 20 eigenfunctions. Figure 3 gives an example of the correspondence map of a pair of trunk surfaces acquired during clinical follow-up. Corresponding points are correctly computed between the deformable shapes and are independent of local and global differences between the surface models.

2.3   Statistical Analysis of Local Deformations

The correspondence map c (Sect. 2.2) enables accurate point-wise comparison between local features of shapes. To do this, let us consider two feature vectors $\mathbf{F}$ and $\mathbf{G}$ on meshes M_1 and M_2, respectively. Here, M_1 and M_2 belong to same individual and are measured at different time points. Our feature vector represents the geometric information of the mesh, as for instance surface point (depth) coordinates, i.e. $F(\mathbf{x}) = (x, y, z)^T$. A point-wise comparison between M_1 and M_2 can then be established from the l_2 difference of their multivariate features: $\delta(\mathbf{x}) = \|F(\mathbf{x}) - G(c(\mathbf{x}))\|^2$, at each point $\mathbf{x}$ and for a given point mapping c. This means that we could simply test the statistical significance of the difference between feature components at the corresponding vertex pairs in M_1 and M_2. However, the test statistic obtained by the simple difference would ignore the inherent correlation between deformable shapes, and consequently, would be less sensitive to small changes. Indeed, longitudinally sampled scoliotic trunks are highly correlated when the scoliosis progresses moderately; changes in the shape deformities will therefore have very small amplitudes. One possible solution is to weight the feature vectors so that their statistical differences become significantly high. We therefore propose to combine the correspondence map with CCA [11].

Canonical Correlation Analysis (CCA) with Correspondence. The principle of CCA is to find a linear transformation that captures the relationship between two groups of multivariate vectors. Given two groups of features $\mathbf{F}$ and $\mathbf{G}$ (of n dimensions) at corresponding vertices, the canonical correlation finds, simultaneously, the weight matrices $\mathbf{a} = (a_1, ..., a_n)$ and $\mathbf{b} = (b_1, ..., b_n)$ whose column vectors are ordered w.r.t. the degree of positive correlation between $\mathbf{F}$ and $\mathbf{G}$— first canonical variates $(a_1^T \mathbf{F}, b_1^T \mathbf{G})$ are the linear combinations with the largest correlation—and the variances $\mathrm{Var}[\mathbf{a}^T \mathbf{F}]$, $\mathrm{Var}[\mathbf{b}^T \mathbf{G}]$ are equal to one. This normalization constraint ensures a uniform scaling of all the features, and therefore ensures that we get unique weight coefficients for all the corresponding points.

Our strategy is then to establish a point-wise comparison from the differences between canonical variates having maximal variance. This is analogous to finding the linear combinations with minimal (non-negative) correlation [16,17], since

$$\mathrm{Var}\{\mathbf{a}^T \mathbf{F} - \mathbf{b}^T \mathbf{G}\} = 2(1 - \mathrm{Corr}[\mathbf{a}^T \mathbf{F}, \mathbf{b}^T \mathbf{G}]). \tag{4}$$

Accordingly, differences with maximal variance are obtained by reversing the correlation order between canonical variates so that the first difference component refers to the highest variance. Point-wise comparison is consequently established between a set of canonical variates $\mathbf{a}^T \mathbf{F}$, $\mathbf{b}^T \mathbf{G}$ as follows

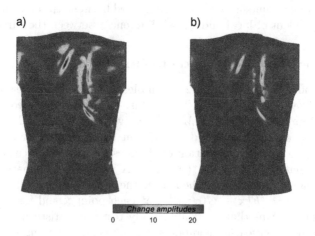

Fig. 4. Statistical change maps for a deformable scoliotic trunk shape using (a) the l_2 differences between transformed features (normal vector coordinates) with the CCA, and (b) the direct l_2 differences.

$$\delta(\mathbf{x}) = \sum_{k=1}^{m} \frac{(a_{n-k+1}^T F(\mathbf{x}) - b_{n-k+1}^T G(c(\mathbf{x})))^2}{v_{n-k+1}}, \ \mathbf{x} \in M_1 \tag{5}$$

where v_k is the k-th component of the variance obtained from Eq. (4). Please note that all the difference components are mutually independent. Furthermore, the linear transformation given by the CCA allows the difference components between canonical variates to approximate zero-mean normal distributions [17] at each corresponding point. Therefore, the difference measure in Eq. (5) defines the $\chi^2(m)$ test statistic with $m \leq n$ degrees of freedom. (In our application, $n = 3$, and m is set to be equal to n.) Figure 4 shows one example of how the CCA transformation can improve the power of the test statistic relative to the direct l_2 difference between matching features.

3   Results and Discussion

Our method was evaluated on 23 scoliotic patients aged 10–18 years having a right thoracic curvature in the normal spine. All the subjects were scanned at an initial visit ($t = 0$) and at 6 and 12 months from their first visit. The trunk surface meshes contained 40k to 70k vertices according to the size of the patient. The trunk model was cropped off at the arms, neck and pelvis using standard control points. These consisted of the left and right points at the corners of the acromions and of 4 anatomical landmarks located manually by an technician by palpation at the following locations: left and right anterior-superior iliac spines (ASIS), midpoint of the posterior-superior iliac spines (MPSIS) and C7 vertebral prominence (VP) [22]. The mesh boundaries were subsequently removed by interpolation (Sect. 2.1). This pre-processing step ensured that holes were filled and noise was reduced at the cropped regions. The spectral correspondence was computed by matching within-subject meshes to a template, the latter defined at the initial visit, to ensure accurate vertex-wise feature comparison across all time points. For feature comparison, we locally approximated the mesh by its tangent plane, orthogonal to the normal vector, at each point $F(\mathbf{x}) = (nx, ny, nz)^T$. We then used the CCA method to capture the differences between the local features, defined as the normal vectors, between pairs of meshes at corresponding vertices. Figure 5 shows the result of our method (spectral correspondence with CCA) for two trunk shapes at 0 and 6 months intervals for a patient who was clinically assessed with a progressive scoliosis between these successive visits. Feature vectors $\mathbf{F}$ of the first mesh (M_1) and their correspondence ($\mathbf{G}$) on the second mesh M_2 are illustrated at each vertex on M_1 for visual comparison. Significant changes in the trunk shape are indicated as the black regions on the detection map. These were identified using CCA with a $p < 0.05$ significance test.

We evaluated our method quantitatively by comparing the trunk shape changes across time to the increase of the Cobb angle (CA), a standard clinical index which measures the curvature of the spine as acquired in a radiographic image (in degrees). We therefore computed the normalized local surface area

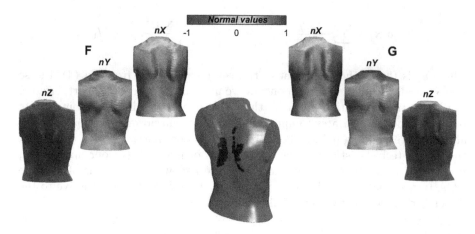

Fig. 5. Statistical analysis of local shape deformations for assessment of SP. Shown here are within-subject scoliotic trunks scanned at 0 and 6 months intervals, with a progressive thoracic spinal curve (15° increase of Cobb angle). Feature vectors **F** and **G** are represented at corresponding points on the template surface (scanned at 0 months interval). Our method reveals 3% of significant changes (in terms of the normalized local surface area) in regions located on the back (*in black on the detection map at the center*) at 5% test of significance. (Color figure online)

(in percentage) of the changes in trunk deformations during the follow-up; the local surface area of the longitudinal changes is normalized w.r.t. the total surface area of the subject's template (acquisition at $t = 0$). This normalization compensates for the different torso sizes across the population. Table 1 summarizes the CA statistics for all 23 patients as well as the averages for the progressive and non-progressive groups. For clinical purposes, a scoliosis case is considered progressive when the measured CA increases by 6° or more between 2 acquisitions. Table 2 illustrates the confusion matrix between our method and the ground truth data. This comparison shows that all 7 patients clinically evaluated as progressive had significant trunk shape changes across the two follow-up time points using our method. The average increase of the normalized area of scoliotic deformities was $(2.7 \pm 1.8)\%$, whereas the average increase in CA across this group was 9°. This means that for this group of patients, whose spinal deviations progressed moderately, the proposed method was able to capture, on average, 2.7% change in the shape deformations associated with SP. Moreover, significant shape changes were detected in 4 out of 16 non-progressive scoliotic patients. These cases are reported as false positives with respect to the ground truth clinical assessment. They are mainly due to outliers located at the cropped boundaries of the trunk. The uncertainty in the placement of the anatomic landmarks leads to variability in the cropping of the trunk model and therefore to uncertainty errors in matching the boundary regions. On the other hand, SP is evaluated clinically solely on the basis of deviations of the spine through CA measurement. But the CA remains limited to assessing the spinal deformity in a 2D radiographic projection, while the shape of the scoliotic trunk is also affected

Table 1. Summary CA statistics for 23 scoliotic trunks characterized by a right thoracic spinal curve (in degrees).

t (mo)	Max	Mean	SD	Mean of progressive group	Mean of non-progressive group
0	47	21	18	37	15
6	58	28	20	46	22
12	59	29	21	51	22

Table 2. Confusion matrix for categorization of patients as progressive or non-progressive: our method versus standard clinical method based on CA.

		Ground truth measurements (CA)	
		Progressive	Non-progressive
Proposed method	Change	7	4
	No change	0	12
Total		7	16

by other factors, in particular the deformation of the rib cage (manifested as a hump at the back). This latter deformation is caused by the axial rotation of vertebrae [10]. Figure 6 shows one case of a follow-up patient whose scoliosis was considered non-progressive according to the CA, while a hump at the back progressed significantly between the 6 and 12 month time points. This is considered as a false positive according to the CA assessment. Rib hump deformation is in fact one of the first diagnostic indicators of scoliosis, in particular during its early stages; it is also one of the most visible signs affecting the cosmetic appearance of the trunk, which is the major concern of young patients [5,23]. Our preliminary results demonstrate the importance and the effectiveness of including longitudinal shape analysis in scoliosis assessment routines. We aim to strengthen these results by means of larger datasets and more extensive validation. Moreover, in order to efficiently evaluate SP, we excluded in this work all possible changes on the anterior side of the trunk. These changes, particularly observed in young female patients, are affected by the deformation of the chest, which might be due to different factors: asymmetry changes associated with scoliosis, position of the arms or growth; they might therefore lead to ambiguity in SP assessment. Even with a standardized positioning of the arms, the morphological correlation between the normal anatomical changes of the body (e.g., body fat and growth) and scoliosis deformations prompted us to focus on the posterior side of the trunk. Analysis of full-torso changes would require an evaluation of the normal variability of scoliotic trunk shapes during the anatomical development of adolescents.

Finally, we evaluated the performance of the point-wise statistical analysis using the CCA transformation of shape features against direct comparison, i.e., simple point-wise differences (Sect. 2.3). For this evaluation, we compared the increase in the normalized local surface area of the trunk deformations during

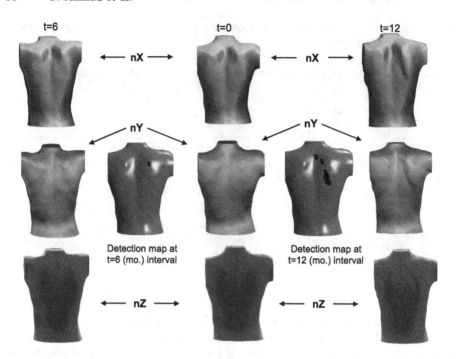

Fig. 6. One progressive case considered as a false positive compared to the CA ground truth. Middle column: feature vector (normal vector coordinates $\mathbf{F}(\mathbf{x}) = (nx, ny, nz)$) of the scoliotic trunk at the initial visit ($t = 0$ mo. interval). Left and right columns: shape features at $t = 6$ and $t = 12$ mo. intervals, respectively. Detection maps are obtained using spectral correspondence to $t = 0$ and CCA for 5% test of significance.

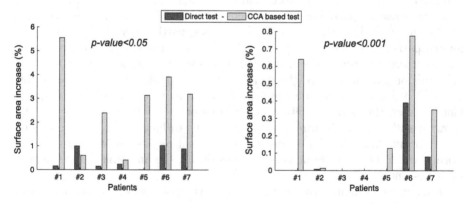

Fig. 7. Performance of the statistical analysis using CCA transformation of matching features versus direct comparison, for the follow-up of 7 progressive cases. The CCA significantly improves the test statistic for both $p < 0.05$ and $p < 0.001$.

the follow-up of the 7 patients having progressive scoliosis. Figure 7 shows that the CCA significantly improves the detection power of the χ^2 test statistic (for $p < 0.05$ and $p < 0.001$). On average, a 2.74% increase in the surface area is detected by the CCA method for $p < 0.05$, and 3.22% for $p < 0.001$, while the test using direct comparison detects only very small areas of change in the shape deformities (0.5% for $p < 0.05$ and 0.08% for $p < 0.001$). Further research could investigate whether a statistical model [2] that considers the spatial relationship between each vertex and its neighborhood can improve the underlying point-wise statistical analysis.

4 Conclusion

In this contribution, we addressed longitudinal shape analysis of scoliotic trunks using a spectral representation of surface models and point-wise feature comparison via CCA. The main originality of our work is the spectral representation and the efficient computation of shape correspondences in order to compare different scoliotic trunks over time. For the first time, scoliotic trunk analysis is based on the spectral representation of shapes. However, correct shape correspondence remains a challenging problem in our context because of the variability between acquisitions in the cropping of the surface models at the trunk boundaries. Future work will focus on this issue. In our validation study, we considered a single type of scoliotic deformation to test the performance of our method against the standard evaluation based on Cobb angles. Quantitive comparison with the clinical ground truth demonstrates the effectiveness of our shape analysis method for scoliosis follow-up and progression assessment.

Future work will be threefold: we will focus on the issue of shape matching in the presence of uncertainty at the trunk boundaries; we will consider larger patient sets including several scoliotic deformation types for validation; finally, we will look at adapting this framework for other applications such as predicting scoliosis progression and evaluating the effect of spine correction on trunk asymmetry.

Acknowledgments. This research was funded by the Canadian Institutes of Health Research (grant number MPO 125875). The authors would like to thank Philippe Debanné for revising this paper and the anonymous reviewers for their insightful comments and suggestions.

References

1. Adankon, M.M., Chihab, N., Dansereau, J., Labelle, H., Cheriet, F.: Scoliosis follow-up using noninvasive trunk surface acquisition. IEEE Trans. Biomed. Eng. **60**(8), 2262–2270 (2013)
2. Ahmad, O., Collet, C.: Scale-space spatio-temporal random fields: application to the detection of growing microbial patterns from surface roughness. Pattern Recogn. **58**, 27–38 (2016)

3. Ajemba, P.O., Durdle, N.G., Raso, V.J.: Characterizing torso shape deformity in scoliosis using structured splines models. IEEE Trans. Biomed. Eng. **56**(6), 1652–1662 (2009)
4. Belkin, M., Niyogi, P.: Laplacian eigenmaps for dimensionality reduction and data representation. Neural Comput. **15**(6), 1373–1396 (2003)
5. Buchanan, R., Birch, J.G., Morton, A.A., Browne, R.H.: Do you see what I see? Looking at scoliosis surgical outcomes through orthopedists' eyes. Spine **28**(24), 2700–2704 (2003). discussion 2705
6. Carr, J.C., Beatson, R.K., Cherrie, J.B., Mitchell, T.J., Fright, W.R., McCallum, B.C., Evans, T.R.: Reconstruction and representation of 3D objects with radial basis functions. In: Proceedings of the 28th Annual Conference on Computer Graphics and Interactive Techniques, SIGGRAPH 2001, pp. 67–76. ACM, New York (2001)
7. Cobb, J.R.: Outline for the study of scoliosis. Am. Acad. Orthop. Surg. Instruct. Lect. **5**, 261–275 (1984)
8. Fischl, B., Sereno, M.I., Tootell, R.B., Dale, A.M.: High-resolution intersubject averaging and a coordinate system for the cortical surface. Hum. Brain Mapp. **8**(4), 272–284 (1999)
9. Grigis, A., Noblet, V., Heitz, F., Blanc, F., de Sèze, J., Kremer, S., Rumbach, L., Armspach, J.P.: Longitudinal change detection in diffusion MRI using multivariate statistical testing on tensors. NeuroImage **60**(4), 2206–2221 (2012)
10. Hackenberg, L., Hierholzer, E., Pötzl, W., Götze, C., Liljenqvist, U.: Rasterstereographic back shape analysis in idiopathic scoliosis after posterior correction and fusion. Clin. Biomech. **18**(10), 883–889 (2003)
11. Hotelling, H.: Relations between two sets of variates. Biometrika **XXVIII**, 321–377 (1936)
12. Jain, V., Zhang, H.: Robust 3D shape correspondence in the spectral domain. In: IEEE International Conference on Shape Modeling and Applications 2006 (SMI 2006), p. 19, June 2006
13. Lombaert, H., Grady, L., Polimeni, J.R., Cheriet, F.: FOCUSR: feature oriented correspondence using spectral regularization-a method for precise surface matching. IEEE Trans. Pattern Anal. Mach. Intell. **35**(9), 2143–2160 (2013)
14. Lombaert, H., Arcaro, M., Ayache, N.: Brain transfer: spectral analysis of cortical surfaces and functional maps. Inf. Process. Med. Imaging **24**, 474–487 (2015)
15. Lombaert, H., Grady, L., Pennec, X., Ayache, N., Cheriet, F.: Spectral demons-image registration via global spectral correspondence. In: Fitzgibbon, A., Lazebnik, S., Perona, P., Sato, Y., Schmid, C. (eds.) Computer Vision - ECCV 2012. LNCS, vol. 7573, pp. 30–44. Springer, Heidelberg (2012)
16. Nielsen, A.: The regularized iteratively reweighted MAD method for change detection in multi- and hyperspectral data. IEEE Trans. Image Process. **16**(2), 463–478 (2007)
17. Nielsen, A.A., Conradsen, K., Simpson, J.J.: Multivariate alteration detection (MAD) and MAF postprocessing in multispectral, bitemporal image data: new approaches to change detection studies. remote Sens. Environ. **64**(1), 1–19 (1998)
18. Pazos, V., Cheriet, F., Danserau, J., Ronsky, J., Zernicke, R.F., Labelle, H.: Reliability of trunk shape measurements based on 3-D surface reconstructions. Eur. Spine J. **16**(11), 1882–1891 (2007)
19. Reuter, M.: Hierarchical shape segmentation and registration via topological features of laplace-Beltrami eigenfunctions. Int. J. Comput. Vis. **89**(2–3), 287–308 (2009)

20. Reuter, M., Wolter, F.E., Peinecke, N.: Laplace-spectra as fingerprints for shape matching. In: Proceedings of the 2005 ACM Symposium on Solid and Physical Modeling, SPM 2005, pp. 101–106. ACM, New York (2005)
21. Richards, B.S., Bernstein, R.M., D'Amato, C.R., Thompson, G.H.: Standardization of criteria for adolescent idiopathic scoliosis brace studies: SRS committee on bracing and nonoperative management. Spine **30**(18), 2068–2075 (2005). Discussion 2076–2077
22. Seoud, L., Dansereau, J., Labelle, H., Cheriet, F.: Multilevel analysis of trunk surface measurements for noninvasive assessment of scoliosis deformities. Spine **37**(17), E1045–E1053 (2012)
23. Tones, M., Moss, N., Polly, D.W.: A review of quality of life and psychosocial issues in scoliosis. Spine **31**(26), 3027–3038 (2006)

Statistical Shape Model with Random Walks for Inner Ear Segmentation

Esmeralda Ruiz Pujadas[1(✉)], Hans Martin Kjer[2], Gemma Piella[1], and Miguel Angel González Ballester[1,3]

[1] Department of Information and Communication Technologies,
Universitat Pompeu Fabra, 08018 Barcelona, Spain
`esmeralda.ruiz@upf.edu`
[2] Department of Applied Mathematics and Computer Science,
Technical University of Denmark, Lyngby, Denmark
[3] ICREA, Barcelona, Spain

Abstract. Cochlear implants can restore hearing to completely or partially deaf patients. The intervention planning can be aided by providing a patient-specific model of the inner ear. Such a model has to be built from high resolution images with accurate segmentations. Thus, a precise segmentation is required. We propose a new framework for segmentation of micro-CT cochlear images using random walks combined with a statistical shape model (SSM). The SSM allows us to constrain the less contrasted areas and ensures valid inner ear shape outputs. Additionally, a topology preservation method is proposed to avoid the leakage in the regions with no contrast.

Keywords: Random walks · Segmentation · Shape prior · Iterative segmentation · Distance map prior · Statistical shape model · SSM · Cochlea segmentation · Inner ear segmentation

1 Introduction

The HEAR-EU[1] project aims at reducing the inter-patient variability in the outcomes of surgical electrode implantation by improving CI designs and surgical protocols using computational models [1,2]. These models are generally built from the segmentations of high resolution images where a large amount of intra-cochlear structures are visible on the image. In this context, we propose a method that enables an accurate segmentation of the inner ear in micro-CT images which contains the hearing organ known as the cochlea. This aids the generation of accurate patient-specific computational models, which can guide implant design, insertion planning and selection of the best treatment strategy for each patient.

The research leading to these results received funding from the European Union Seventh Frame Programme (FP7/2007-2013) under grant agreement 304857.

[1] http://www.hear-eu.eu/.

© Springer International Publishing AG 2016
M. Reuter et al. (Eds.): SeSAMI 2016, LNCS 10126, pp. 92–102, 2016.
DOI: 10.1007/978-3-319-51237-2_8

There are a few studies on semi- or fully automatic inner ear segmentation from micro-CT data. However, due to the complexity of the anatomical structure, it is generally a manual procedure [3]. One semi-automatic approach to obtain the cochlea is based on 2D snakes [4], but it requires a high degree of user interaction to locate the initial contour and adjustment of the parameters. Another technique is based on statistical shape models (SSMs) [5], where the high resolution segmentations are used to build a statistical model and assist the segmentation of low resolution cochlear images. In order to accurately segment the cochlea in high resolution micro-CT images using the classical SSM approach introduced by Cootes [6], a large number of processed data sets would be required to learn the correct anatomical variability of the data. The scarce availability of micro-CT images means that we have to consider other segmentation strategies.

In order to alleviate these issues, we proposed a new algorithm using random walks with a distance-based shape prior, which is robust independently of the chosen prior and which requires no user interaction [7,8]. Random walks segmentation is a graph-based segmentation method proposed by Grady [9]. This technique has become very popular because it is robust to noise and weak boundaries and it can be easily extended to 3D and to an arbitrary number of labels. According to the author, random walks can outperform the well-known graph cuts [10] in terms of weak boundaries since the latter tries to minimize the total edge weights in the cut. Thus, graph cuts may return very small segmentations ("small cut" behaviour) in presence of low contrast, a small number of seeds or noise [9]. Additionally, random walks can be straightforwardly generalized to multi-label segmentation unlike graph cuts which usually use complex alpha-beta techniques [11].

Generally, the intensity information is not enough to obtain the object of interest. Thus, a shape prior can be incorporated to be able to separate the target object from the rest of the image. Some techniques to incorporate prior knowledge into random walks have been proposed. Constrained random walks algorithm is developed for pedestrian segmentation [12]. Given binary pedestrian silhouette images as a training data, a pedestrian shape prior model is built by averaging the training data for every pose, as well as averaging all training data to obtain a general prior model. The pedestrian shape models are incorporated into the random walks formulation. The constrained random walks are applied for every shape model separately, and the final segmentation is the one with the highest probability. Baudin et al. proposed a similar work applied to the skeletal muscle [13]. The prior model of the thigh muscles is derived from learning a Gaussian model based on previous segmentations of the thigh muscles in a training set. The main drawback of both methods is the sensitivity to the average model and to the registration inaccuracies. The same may occur in [14] where prior knowledge is obtained from a probabilistic atlas to perform prostate segmentation. In order to allow large scale deformations, Baudin et al. introduced the principal component analysis (PCA) into the random walks formulation [15]. The shape deformation is constrained to remain close to PCA shape space built from training examples. However, the method does not allow representing shapes that differ too much from the standard shapes [16]. According to the authors, PCA can not deal properly with probabilities. Thus, they suggest to find a different shape space more compatible with probabilities such as the barycentric model. A similar work using PCA is presented in [17] which utilizes a PCA-based shape model as a prior but it is also sensitive to the average shape. In order not to be constrained to the average shape, the guided random walks are proposed [18] where the closest subject to the target object in a given database is retrieved to guide the segmentation. If there is not a close shape in the database, the standard random walks are performed. The limitations of this method are that all the samples of the training data must be considered in order to find the closest data set to the target image and that in case there is no good match, it only relies on the standard random walks. Random walks with shape prior have also been used for video tracking and segmentation [19,20].

An extension of random walks was presented by Grady in [21] by integrating a non-parametric probability density model which allows localization of disconnected objects and eliminates the requirement of user-specified labels. We use this framework to incorporate prior knowledge into random walks formulation where the region term and the shape prior information given by a SSM constitute the probability density model.

There are some works combining a classical segmentation method with a SSM. Two of the most common methods are based on graph cuts [22–28] and level sets [29–32] where they generally use an implicit representation of shapes such as a signed distance map relaxing the need for a costly landmark detection and matching process. In our work, we choose random walks due to the numerous advantages mentioned above.

In this paper, we present an extension of our previous work [7,8] combining random walks with a SSM to benefit from the strengths of both methods. The region term is combined with a distance-based prior constrained by a SSM. The SSM allows us to constrain the segmentation to a valid inner ear shape to obtain anatomically correct segmentation results. The confidence map adjusts the influence of the prior in certain areas making the method, along with the region term, less sensitive to the average shape. A topology preservation method is also proposed to avoid leakage in the interior and the turns of the cochlea [33]. In the remainder of this paper, we explain the details of the proposed method and show the experimental results on micro-CT images of the inner ear.

2 Random Walks Segmentation

An image can be represented as a graph where the nodes are the pixels of the image, and the weights represent the similarity between nodes. Vertices marked by the user as seeds are denoted by V_m and the rest by V_u. Given some seeds, $v_j \in V_m$, the random walker assigns to each node, $v_i \in V_u$, the probability, x_i^s, that a random walker starting from that node first reaches a marked node, $v_j \in V_m$ assigned to label g^s. The random walks segmentation is then completed by assigning each free node to the label for which it has the highest probability [9].

An extension to random walks was proposed in [21] by incorporating a probability density model based on the gray-level intensity for each label. Let λ_i^s be the probability density that the intensity at node v_i belongs to the intensity distribution of label s. The modified random walks segmentation is obtained by solving the following system [21]:

$$\left(L + \gamma \sum_{r=1}^{n} \Lambda^r\right) x^s = \gamma \lambda^s \tag{1}$$

where $\Lambda = diag(\lambda^s)$, n is the number of labels, γ is a free parameter and L is the Laplacian matrix which can be defined as:

$$L_{ij} = \begin{cases} d_i & \text{if } i = j \\ -w_{ij} & \text{if } v_i \text{ and } v_j \text{ are adjacent nodes} \\ 0 & \text{otherwise} \end{cases} \tag{2}$$

where L_{ij} is indexed by the vertices v_i and v_j and $d_i = \sum_{j=1}^{n} w_{ij}$. The weight function w_{ij} can be computed as:

$$w_{ij} = \exp(-\beta(I_i - I_j)^2) \tag{3}$$

where I_i is the intensity at pixel i and β is a free parameter related to the bandwidth kernel. The weight range is between 0 and 1 and the higher the weight the larger the similarity between pixels [34,35].

For more details, we refer to [21]. In this work, we use this framework to perform image segmentation but instead of using an intensity-based distribution, we propose a more robust density estimation considering region information as well as shape prior knowledge given by a SSM. We explain them in detail in the remaining part of the section.

2.1   Region Term Formulation

The region term partitions the image in terms of intensities (bright versus dark). A histogram is built from one of the slices of the inner ear. Then, two Gaussian components representing the inner ear including other regions with the same intensity profile and the background are fitted to the histogram with a Gaussian mixture model (GMM). The region-based term can be defined as:

$$D_i(l_i) = \begin{cases} -\ln p(x_i|O) & \text{if } l_i = object \\ -\ln p(x_i|B) & \text{if } l_i = background \end{cases} \tag{4}$$

where x_i is the pixel indexed by i, l is the label and $p(x_i|O)$ and $p(x_i|B)$ are the probabilities estimated by the GMM of pixel at i belonging to object and background intensity, respectively.

2.2   Shape Prior Knowledge and Statistical Shape Model

Once the region term is obtained, the shape prior is computed to discard areas which do not belong to the inner ear and have similar intensity values. The use of a SSM can provide a realistic prior to initialize the whole segmentation process, and further be a source of plausible shape regularization during each iteration of the random walker. The SSM is used with a procedure, which we refer to as statistical non-rigid registration, described as follows. We perform a non-rigid image registration between a reference data set, I_R, and the target image, I_S, which in the framework of elastix [36] is formulated as an optimization problem. The (parametric) transformation that aligns the two images, $T_\eta : I_R \to I_S$ is described by the vector η containing q-parameters which is found by optimization of a cost function, $\mathcal{C}$.

$$\hat{\eta} = \arg \min_{\eta} \mathcal{C}(T_\eta^{SDM}, I_R, I_S), \text{ where } \mathcal{C} = \mathcal{S}_{\mathrm{Sim}}(\eta, I_R, I_S) \tag{5}$$

The chosen transformation is a B-Spline model regularized by a Statistical Deformation Model (SDM) to constrain the non-rigid registration. The SDM was trained by registering a reference data set against 16 different data sets using the registration model described in [37]. The output of each registration is a vector of q-deformation parameters which describes a B-Spline deformation field. Considering the parameters of the B-Spline model to be corresponding variables, a principal component analysis on the 16 fields was made using Statismo [38] to obtain a description of deformation variability in a reduced parameter-space. This type of transformation model is made available through an integration of the Statismo-elastix packages. The cost function, $\mathcal{C}$, is solely an image similarity measure, in this case using the normalized correlation coefficient. Note, that if the image intensities were normalized to the HU scale, it would be sufficient to use the sum of squared differences. That was, however, not the case for our data. The optimization is solved using Adaptive Stochastic Gradient Descent [39], which is shown to be a good choice for medical image registration with a limited number of parameters [36,39].

From the statistical non-rigid registration, the deformation between the reference and target images is applied to the segmentation of the reference data set to obtain the shape prior. This prior is constrained to be an anatomically correct cochlea and from its contour we can build a distance map. The idea is that given an estimation of the location and shape of the object to segment, pixels close to the shape contour are more likely to be labelled as foreground and vice versa. The formulation can be defined as follows [40]:

$$S_i(l_i = object, \theta) = p(x_i = object|\Theta) = 1 - p(x_i = background|\Theta) = \frac{1}{1 + \exp(\mu \cdot (d(i, \Theta) - d_r))} \tag{6}$$

where $d(i, \Theta)$ is the distance of a pixel i from a shape Θ, being negative inside the shape and positive outside the shape. Here, μ is a penalty term determined by the ratio of points outside the shape compared to the points inside the shape and d_r is the "width" of influence of the shape.

Then, the distance-based shape prior term is:

$$S_i(l_i, \Theta) = \begin{cases} p(x = object|\Theta) & \text{if } l_i = object \\ 1 - p(x = object|\Theta) & \text{if } l_i = background \end{cases} \tag{7}$$

2.3 Random Walks with Region and Prior Knowledge Terms

We combine the region and shape prior terms by a weighted sum. We use a confidence map to adjust the influence of the shape prior according to the strength of the image contour by reducing the weight of this prior where strong contours are present. The formulation is as follows:

$$E_{total}(l_i) = kS_i(l_i, \Theta) \cdot c_i + (1 - k)D_i(l_i) \cdot \frac{1}{c_i}. \tag{8}$$

where k is the weight of each term and c is the confidence map defined as $c_i = \exp(-k_v \sigma_r^2(i))$ where $\sigma_r^2(i)$ is the variance at pixel i computed on a patch with radius r, and k_v is a free parameter that determines the bandwidth of the Gaussian. Equation 8 is used to obtain λ^s in the random walks formulation in Eq. 1 for every label, which results in a segmentation. This segmentation is statistically non-rigidly registered against the reference segmentation to obtain a new prior constrained by the SSM. Note that this second registration is performed in the binary segmentation in contrast to the initial prior whose registration was between the grayscale reference and target images and the resulting deformation was applied to the reference segmentation to obtain the prior. The distance-based prior is then built from Eq. 6 and the random walks segmentation is performed again. This procedure continues until convergence or until the maximum number of iterations is reached. In order to avoid merging the non-contrasted areas of the cochlea, the topology preserving method described in [33] is proposed. The topology preservation method computes the unit outward normal vector of the contour and when two vectors are pointing in opposite directions, the contours in this area are not allowed to merge.

3 Results

In this experiment, 10 micro-CT data sets of the inner ear are used to perform the segmentation in 3D using the proposed method. The original 3D data set was downsampled from a nominal isotropic resolution of $24.5\,\mu$m to $49\,\mu$m for computational efficiency reasons. Every data set contains around 213 slices with an average size of 413×275 pixels. The ground truth is manually annotated. The initial prior is obtained as described in Sect. 2.2. The SSM is built from 17 different data sets (one reference and 16 training samples).

The following parameters were used to produce the results: $\gamma = 0.8$ in Eq. 1, $d_r = 0$ and $\mu = 1.0$ in Eq. 6 and the total number of iterations are 4 with $k = 0.8$ in Eq. 8.

Some inner ear segmentation results using our approach are illustrated in Fig. 1. In this example, we can observe from the 3D volume that the topology

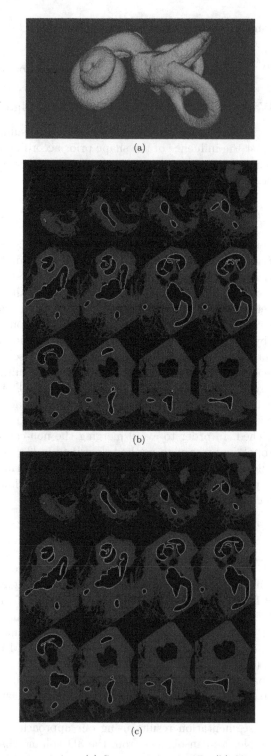

Fig. 1. Inner Ear segmentation. (a) Segmentation in 3D. (b) Slices of the 3D segmentation. (c) Ground truth.

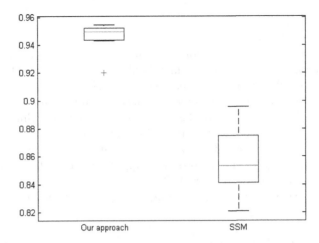

Fig. 2. Segmentation quality shown as a box plot in terms of the Dice similarity coefficient for the proposed approach and the SSM alone. The results of our method show a smaller standard variation and better performance than the other technique.

of the inner ear shape is preserved and that the contour of the segmentation is adjusted to the edges of the image whereas the interior of the cochlea and less contrasted areas are conserved due to the shape prior and topology preservation method.

To quantify the segmentation quality for the proposed method, we compute the well-known Dice with respect to a manual ground truth. The formulation is defined as $Dice = \frac{2TP}{2TP+FN+FP}$ where TP and FP stand for true positive and false positive and TN and FN for true negative and false negative. We compare our approach with the initial shape prior (corresponding to using the SSM alone) described in Sect. 2.2. The proposed method achieves a mean Dice index of 0.947 and the initial shape prior reaches a mean Dice index of 0.856. The reason for a lower value is that 17 samples are obviously not enough to cover the true variability in inner ear shapes in high resolution images. The results are presented in Fig. 2 where we can observe a high improvement from using the SSM alone. In contrast with the SSM method alone, the Dice similarity coefficients computed from the segmentation results of the proposed technique have a smaller standard deviation having a small range of Dice values between [0.94,0.95] except for one single case that it has a 0.92 of Dice. The reason of these satisfactory results is that the exterior of the cochlea can be efficiently separated as there is enough contrast between the cochlea and background and the small and invisible regions can be extracted with the guidance of the prior. The topology preservation method prevents leakage in the non-contrasted areas. In high gradient areas of the image (edges) around the prior, the confidence map reduces the influence of the prior coping with the possible artefacts and inaccuracies in the prior shape. It is clear that for internal regions, this method relies on the prior but the SSM constrains the shape of these areas and for the exterior of the inner ear, the region term with the prior can provide promising results.

4   Conclusion

We presented a new framework for the inner ear segmentation in micro-CT using the random walks algorithm which is able to deal with weak boundaries efficiently. The combination of the distance map prior with a region term into random walks provides accurate segmentations of the inner ear. The SSM allows us to constrain the interior part of the cochlea to a valid shape while the exterior of the contour evolves along the shape prior. In this work, the SSM is implemented as a non-rigid registration with learnt statistical shape regularization. The experiments suggest that the proposed approach is robust and accurate for the inner ear segmentation in micro-CT images. As future work, we would like to do an exhaustive analysis and thorough study of this method as well as a comparison with other methods.

Acknowledgments. The research leading to these results received funding from the European Union Seventh Frame Programme (FP7/2007–2013) under grant agreement 304857, HEAR-EU Project.

References

1. Ceresa, M., et al.: Patient-specific simulation of implant placement and function for cochlear implantation surgery planning. In: Golland, P., Hata, N., Barillot, C., Hornegger, J., Howe, R. (eds.) MICCAI 2014. LNCS, vol. 8674, pp. 49–56. Springer, Heidelberg (2014). doi:10.1007/978-3-319-10470-6_7
2. Ceresa, M., Mangado, N., Andrews, R.J., Ballester, M.A.G.: Computational models for predicting outcomes of neuroprosthesis implantation: the case of cochlear implants. Mol. Neurobiol. **52**(2), 934–941 (2015)
3. Braun, K., Böhnke, F., Stark, T.: Three-dimensional representation of the human cochlea using micro-computed tomography data: presenting an anatomical model for further numerical calculations. Acta Oto-Laryngologica **132**(6), 603–613 (2012)
4. Poznyakovskiy, A.A., Zahnert, T., Kalaidzidis, Y., Lazurashvili, N., Schmidt, R., Hardtke, H.-J., Fischer, B., Yarin, Y.M.: A segmentation method to obtain a complete geometry model of the hearing organ. Hear. Res. **282**(1), 25–34 (2011)
5. Noble, J.H., Labadie, R.F., Majdani, O., Dawant, B.M.: Automatic segmentation of intracochlear anatomy in conventional CT. IEEE Trans. Biomed. Eng. **58**(9), 2625–2632 (2011)
6. Cootes, T.F., Taylor, C.J., Cooper, D.H., Graham, J.: Active shape models-their training and application. Comput. Vis. Image Underst. **61**(1), 38–59 (1995)
7. Pujadas, E.R., Kjer, H.M., Piella, G., Ceresa, M., Ballester, M.A.G.: Random walks with shape prior for cochlea segmentation in ex vivo μCT. Int. J. Comput. Assist. Radiol. Surg. **11**(9), 1647–1659 (2016)
8. Pujadas, E.R., Kjer, H.M., Piella, G., Ballester, M.A.G.: Iterated random walks with shape prior. Image Vis. Comput. **54**, 12–21 (2016)
9. Grady, L.: Random walks for image segmentation. IEEE Trans. Pattern Anal. Mach. Intell. **28**(11), 1768–1783 (2006)
10. Boykov, Y., Veksler, O.: Graph cuts in vision and graphics: theories and applications. In: Paragios, N., Chen, Y., Faugeras, O. (eds.) Handbook of Mathematical Models in Computer Vision, pp. 79–96. Springer, Heidelberg (2006)

11. Boykov, Y., Veksler, O., Zabih, R.: Fast approximate energy minimization via graph cuts. IEEE Trans. Pattern Anal. Mach. Intell. **23**(11), 1222–1239 (2001)
12. Li, K.-C., Su, H.-R., Lai, S.-H.: Pedestrian image segmentation via shape-prior constrained random walks. In: Ho, Y.-S. (ed.) PSIVT 2011. LNCS, vol. 7088, pp. 215–226. Springer, Heidelberg (2011). doi:10.1007/978-3-642-25346-1_20
13. Baudin, P.-Y., Azzabou, N., Carlier, P.G., Paragios, N.: Prior knowledge, random walks and human skeletal muscle segmentation. In: Ayache, N., Delingette, H., Golland, P., Mori, K. (eds.) MICCAI 2012. LNCS, vol. 7510, pp. 569–576. Springer, Heidelberg (2012). doi:10.1007/978-3-642-33415-3_70
14. Li, A., Li, C., Wang, X., Eberl, S., Feng, D.D., Fulham, M.: Automated segmentation of prostate MR images using prior knowledge enhanced random walker. In: 2013 International Conference on Digital Image Computing: Techniques and Applications (DICTA), pp. 1–7. IEEE (2013)
15. Baudin, P.-Y., Azzabou, N., Carlier, P.G., Paragios, N.: Manifold-enhanced segmentation through random walks on linear subspace priors. In: Proceedings of the British Machine Vision Conference (2012)
16. Baudin, P.-Y.: De la segmentation au moyen de graphes d'images de muscles striés squelettiques acquises par RMN. Ph.D. thesis, Ecole Centrale Paris (2013)
17. Ting, Y., Xiaoming Liu, S., Lim, N.K., Tu, P.H.: Automatic surveillance video matting using a shape prior. In: 2011 IEEE International Conference on Computer Vision Workshops (ICCV Workshops), pp. 1761–1768. IEEE (2011)
18. Eslami, A., Karamalis, A., Katouzian, A., Navab, N.: Segmentation by retrieval with guided random walks: application to left ventricle segmentation in MRI. Med. Image Anal. **17**(2), 236–253 (2013)
19. Lee, Y.-T., Te-Feng, S., Hong-Ren, S., Lai, S.-H., Lee, T.-C., Shih, M.-Y.: Human segmentation from video by combining random walks with human shape prior adaption. In: 2013 Asia-Pacific Signal and Information Processing Association Annual Summit and Conference (APSIPA), pp. 1–4. IEEE (2013)
20. Papoutsakis, K.E., Argyros, A.A.: Object tracking and segmentation in a closed loop. In: Bebis, G., et al. (eds.) ISVC 2010. LNCS, vol. 6453, pp. 405–416. Springer, Heidelberg (2010). doi:10.1007/978-3-642-17289-2_39
21. Grady, L.: Multilabel random walker image segmentation using prior models. In: IEEE Computer Society Conference on Computer Vision and Pattern Recognition, CVPR 2005, vol. 1, pp. 763–770. IEEE (2005)
22. Cremers, D., Grady, L.: Statistical priors for efficient combinatorial optimization via graph cuts. In: Leonardis, A., Bischof, H., Pinz, A. (eds.) ECCV 2006. LNCS, vol. 3953, pp. 263–274. Springer, Heidelberg (2006). doi:10.1007/11744078_21
23. Malcolm, J., Rathi, Y., Tannenbaum, A.: Graph cut segmentation with nonlinear shape priors. In: 2007 IEEE International Conference on Image Processing, vol. 4, pp. 365–368. IEEE (2007)
24. Zhu-Jacquot, J., Zabih, R.: Graph cuts segmentation with statistical shape priors for medical images. In: Third International IEEE Conference on Signal-Image Technologies and Internet-Based System, SITIS 2007, pp. 631–635. IEEE (2007)
25. El-Zehiry, N., Elmaghraby, A.: Graph cut based deformable model with statistical shape priors. In: 19th International Conference on Pattern Recognition, ICPR 2008, pp. 1–4. IEEE (2008)
26. Vu, N., Manjunath, B.S.: Shape prior segmentation of multiple objects with graph cuts. In: 2008 IEEE Conference on Computer Vision and Pattern Recognition, CVPR 2008, pp. 1–8. IEEE (2008)

27. Chen, X., Udupa, J.K., Alavi, A., Torigian, D.A.: GC-ASM synergistic integration of graph-cut and active shape model strategies for medical image segmentation. Comput. Vis. Image Underst. **117**(5), 513–524 (2013)
28. Chang, J.C., Chou, T.: Iterative graph cuts for image segmentation with a nonlinear statistical shape prior. J. Math. Imaging Vis. **49**(1), 87–97 (2014)
29. Leventon, M.E., Eric, W., Grimson, L., Faugeras, O.: Statistical shape influence in geodesic active contours. In: 2000 Proceedings of IEEE Conference on Computer Vision and Pattern Recognition, vol. 1, pp. 316–323. IEEE (2000)
30. Tsai, A., Yezzi, A., Wells, W., Tempany, C., Tucker, D., Fan, A., Grimson, W.E., Willsky, A.: A shape-based approach to the segmentation of medical imagery using level sets. IEEE Trans. Med. Imaging **22**(2), 137–154 (2003)
31. Cremers, D.: Dynamical statistical shape priors for level set-based tracking. IEEE Trans. Pattern Anal. Mach. Intell. **28**(8), 1262–1273 (2006)
32. Cremers, D., Rousson, M., Deriche, R.: A review of statistical approaches to level set segmentation: integrating color, texture, motion and shape. Int. J. Comput. Vis. **72**(2), 195–215 (2007)
33. Pujadas, E.R., Kjer, H.M., Vera, S., Ceresa, M., Ballester, M.A.G.: Cochlea segmentation using iterated random walks with shape prior. In: SPIE Medical Imaging, p. 97842U. International Society for Optics and Photonics (2016)
34. Pujadas, E.R., Reisert, M.: Shape-based normalized cuts using spectral relaxation for biomedical segmentation. IEEE Trans. Image Process. **23**(1), 163–170 (2014)
35. Ruiz, E., Reisert, M.: Image segmentation using normalized cuts with multiple priors. In: SPIE Medical Imaging, p. 866937. International Society for Optics and Photonics (2013)
36. Klein, S., Staring, M., Murphy, K., Viergever, M.A., Pluim, J.P.W.: Elastix: a toolbox for intensity-based medical image registration. IEEE Trans. Med. Imaging **29**(1), 196–205 (2010)
37. Kjer, H.M., Fagertun, J., Vera, S., Gil, D., Ballester, M.Á.G., Paulsen, R.R.: Free-form image registration of human cochlear μCT data using skeleton similarity as anatomical prior. Pattern Recogn. Lett. **76**, 76–82 (2015)
38. Lüthi, M., Blanc, R., Albrecht, T., Gass, T., Goksel, O., Büchler, P., Kistler, M., Bousleiman, H., Reyes, M., Cattin, P., Vetter, T.: Statismo - a framework for PCA based statistical models. Insight J. **1**, 1–18 (2012)
39. Klein, S., Pluim, J.P.W., Staring, M., Viergever, M.A.: Adaptive stochastic gradient descent optimisation for image registration. Int. J. Comput. Vis. **81**(3), 227–239 (2009)
40. Kohli, P., Rihan, J., Bray, M., Torr, P.H.S.: Simultaneous segmentation and pose estimation of humans using dynamic graph cuts. Int. J. Comput. Vis. **79**(3), 285–298 (2008)

Volumetric Image Pattern Recognition Using Three-Way Principal Component Analysis

Hayato Itoh[1], Atsushi Imiya[2(✉)], and Tomoya Sakai[3]

[1] School of Advanced Integration Science, Chiba University,
Yayoi-cho 1-33, Inage-ku, Chiba 263-8522, Japan
[2] Institute of Management and Information Technologies, Chiba University,
Yayoi-cho 1-33, Inage-ku, Chiba 263-8522, Japan
imiya@faculty.chiba-u.jp
[3] Graduate School of Engineering, Nagasaki University,
Bunkyo-cho 1-14, Nagasaki 852-8521, Japan

Abstract. The aim of the paper is to develop a relaxed closed form for tensor principal component analysis (PCA) for the recognition, classification, compression and retrieval of volumetric data. The tensor PCA derives the tensor Karhunen-Loève transform which compresses volumetric data, such as organs, cells in organs and microstructures in cells, preserving both the geometric and statistical properties of objects and spatial textures in the space. Furthermore, we numerically clarify that low-pass filtering after applying the multi-dimensional discrete cosine transform (DCT) efficiently approximates the data compression procedure based on tensor PCA. These orthogonal-projection-based data compression methods for three-way data is extracts outline shapes of biomedical objects such as organs and compressed expressions for the interior structures of cells.

1 Introduction

In this paper, we apply three-way principal component analysis (PCA) to volumetric data analysis in biomedical information processing. For three-way PCA, we develop a relaxed closed form of the tensor PCA computation based on Tucker-3 tensor decomposition, although Tucker-3 tensor decomposition [1,2,5] is achieved by solving variational optimisation problems iteratively. Our method solves a system of variational optimisation problems derived from the original Tucker-3 decomposition with the orthogonal constraints for solutions. This method is used for compression and retrieval of volumetric data preserving volumetric structure with the spatial geometric and statistical properties of shapes [6,8], such as outer boundary of organs, and interior textures of organs, respectively.

Furthermore, these orthogonal-projection-based data compression methods for three-way data arrays extract outline volumetric shapes [7]. Mathematically, a shape is a finite closed region in a Euclidean space. The boundaries of planar and volumetric shapes are closed simple planar curve and closed simple two-dimensional manifolds, respectively. An outline shape is a smoothed profile of

© Springer International Publishing AG 2016
M. Reuter et al. (Eds.): SeSAMI 2016, LNCS 10126, pp. 103–117, 2016.
DOI: 10.1007/978-3-319-51237-2_9

a shape. For a planar shape, an outline shape is generated by smoothing the boundary contour of the shape. For a volumetric shape, an outline shape is generated by smoothing the closed boundary manifold of the shape. These properties imply that outline shapes are generated as smoothed approximations of the original shapes. Outline shapes of volumetric images of organs provide fundamental features for information filtering in medical diagnosis and data retrieval. Furthermore, if a shape is expressed as a series expansion using base functions, an outline of the shape is a finite truncation of this series expansion of the shape. This paper introduces a basis system which simultaneously extracts both outline shape of an object and global statistical properties of interior texture of objects.

Organs, cells in organs and microstructures in cells, which are dealt with in biomedical image analysis, possess statistical properties as spatial textures. These biological objects also possess volumetric structures with spatial geometric and topological properties in the forms of three-dimensional objects [4, 9–12]. Although their local volumetric structures as are computed from geometric and topological properties, their textures estimate both local and global statistical properties of these objects. Organs are essentially spatial textures defined in finite regions. Since these finite regions are organs, the outer boundaries of these regions define the shapes of the organs. For the data analysis of these volumetric data, methods which simultaneously process geometrical and topological structures and spatial texture properties are required.

A pattern is assumed to be a square integrable function in a linear space and to be defined on a finite support in n-dimensional Euclidean space [13]. For planar and volumetric patterns, the dimensions of the Euclidean spaces are two and three, respectively. For the achievement of pattern recognition by numerical computation, sampled patterns are dealt with. In traditional pattern recognition, these sampled patterns are embedded in an appropriate-dimensional Euclidean space as vectors. The other way to deal with sampled patterns is three-way array data. These three-way array data are expressed as tensors [1–3] to preserve the linearity of the original pattern space, since tensors expresses three-way array data in multilinear forms. Therefore, three-way PCA of tensor data extracts features from three-dimensional objects for pattern recognition, classification, compression and data retrieval.

We also numerically clarify that data compression by the discrete cosine transform (DCT) [16] efficiently approximates the data compression procedure based on tensor PCA, since the DCT approximates the Karhunen-Loève (K-L) transform [14, 15].

2   Tensor Analysis and Sampling

Functions and Tensors. For $x \in \mathbb{R}^3$ and $X \in \mathbb{R}^{m \times n}$, $|x|_2$ and $|X|_F$ are the vector norm and Frobenius norm of x and X, respectively. For L_2, W_{21} and W_{22}, the norms are defined as

$$|f|_2 = \left(\int_{\mathbb{R}^3} |f|^2 x \right)^{\frac{1}{2}},$$

$$(1)$$

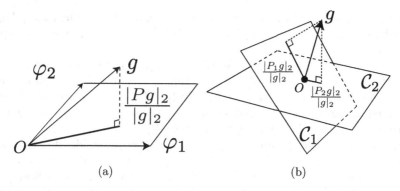

Fig. 1. Subspace method. (a) Setting φ_1 and φ_2 to be the basis of a linear subspace corresponding to a pattern, for an input g, the similarity between g and a pattern in a pattern space is measured by the length of the orthogonal projection of g to the pattern space. (b) Setting P_1 and P_2 to be operators for subspaces $\mathcal{C}_1$ and $\mathcal{C}_2$, respectively, the input g is labelled as being in the first class, since the length of the orthogonal projection of g to $\mathcal{C}_1$ is longer than the length of the orthogonal projection of g to $\mathcal{C}_2$.

$$|f|_{21} = \left(\int_{\mathbb{R}^3} (|f|^2 + |\nabla f|^2) d\boldsymbol{x} \right)^{\frac{1}{2}}, \tag{2}$$

$$|f|_{22} = \left(\int_{\mathbb{R}^3} (|f(\boldsymbol{x})|^2 + |\nabla f|^2 + |\nabla\nabla^\top f|_F^2) d\boldsymbol{x} \right)^{\frac{1}{2}}, \tag{3}$$

where ∇f and $\nabla\nabla^\top f$ are the gradient and the Hessian matrix of f, respectively.

Setting $\boldsymbol{\delta}$ and ε to be a small vector and a small positive number, respectively, we have the relation

$$|f(\boldsymbol{x}+\boldsymbol{\delta}) - (f(\boldsymbol{x}) + \boldsymbol{\delta}^\top \nabla f + \frac{1}{2}\boldsymbol{\delta}^\top (\nabla\nabla^\top f)\boldsymbol{\delta})| < \varepsilon, \tag{4}$$

for local geometric perturbations. f, f_x, f_y, f_z, f_{xx}, f_{yy}, f_{zz}, f_{xy}, f_{yz} and f_{zx} are all independent, if f is not sinusoidal in each direction. Therefore, Eq. (4) implies that, for a pattern defined on three-dimensional Euclidean space, the local dimensions of a pattern are four and ten if local geometric perturbations and local bending deformation of the pattern are assumed as local transformations to the pattern.

Figure 1(a) and (b) show geometric properties of the subspace method and multiclass recognition using the subspace method, respectively. Let φ_1 and φ_2 be the basis of a linear subspace for a pattern. For an input g, the similarity is computed using the length of the orthogonal projection of g to the pattern space. The subspace method allows us to achieve multiclass recognition using the orthogonal projections. Setting P_1 and P_2 to be the orthogonal projection operator to subspaces $\mathcal{C}_1$ and $\mathcal{C}_2$, respectively, the input g is recognised as an element in first class, since the length of the orthogonal projection of g to $\mathcal{C}_1$ is longer than the length of the orthogonal projection of g to $\mathcal{C}_2$. The ratio $|Pg|/|g|$ is called the cumulative contribution ratio (CCR) of g to the linear subspace defined by P.

For the triplet of positive integers I_1, I_2 and I_3, the third-order tensor $\mathbb{R}^{I_1 \times I_2 \times I_3}$ is expressed as $\mathcal{X} = ((x_{ijk}))$ Indices i, j and k are called the 1-mode, 2-mode and 3-mode of $\mathcal{X}$, respectively. The tensor space $\mathbb{R}^{I_1 \times I_2 \times I_3}$ is interpreted as the Kronecker product of three vector spaces $\mathbb{R}^{I_1}$, $\mathbb{R}^{I_2}$ and $\mathbb{R}^{I_3}$ such that $\mathbb{R}^{I_1} \otimes \mathbb{R}^{I_2} \otimes \mathbb{R}^{I_3}$. We set $I = \max(I_1, I_2, I_3)$.

For a square integrable function $f(\boldsymbol{x})$, which is zero outside of a finite support Ω in three-dimensional Euclidean space, the sample $Sf(\Delta\boldsymbol{z})$ for $\boldsymbol{z} \in \mathbf{Z}^3$ and $|\boldsymbol{z}|_\infty \leq I$ defines an $I \times I \times I$ three-way array $\mathbf{F}$. To preserve the multi-linearity of the function $f(\boldsymbol{x})$, we deal with the array $\mathbf{F}$ as a third-order tensor $\mathcal{F}$. The operation $vec\mathcal{F}$ derives a vector $\boldsymbol{f} \in \mathbb{R}^{I_{123}}$ for $I_{123} = I_2 \cdot I_2 \cdot I_3$. We can reconstruct f from $\mathcal{F}$ using an interpolation procedure. Figure 2(a) shows the relations among sampled data and multi-way data Fig. 2(b) shows a data compression procedure for multi-way data.

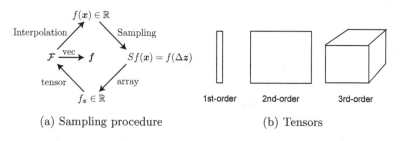

(a) Sampling procedure   (b) Tensors

Fig. 2. Sampling and tensor expression of multi-way data. We can reconstruct f from $\mathcal{F}$ using an interpolation procedure. (a) Shows relations among sampled data and multi-way data. The sampled values of a multivariate function derives multi-way array data. This multi-way array date are dealt with as a higher-order tensor to preserve the multilinear properties of the data. (b) Shows a data compression procedure for multi-way data by deriving a small-size tensor from the original one.

For the outer product of N vectors, if the tensor $\mathcal{X}$ satisfies the condition

$$\mathcal{X} = \boldsymbol{u}^{(1)} \circ \boldsymbol{u}^{(2)} \circ \boldsymbol{u}^{(3)}, \tag{5}$$

where $\circ$ denotes the outer product, we call this tensor $\mathcal{X}$ a rank-one tensor. For $\mathcal{X}$, the n-mode vectors, $n = 1, 2, 3$, are defined as the I_n-dimensional vectors obtained from $\mathcal{X}$ by varying this index i_n while fixing all the other indices.

The unfolding of $\mathcal{X}$ along the n-mode vectors of $\mathcal{X}$ is defined as matrices such that

$$\mathcal{X}_{(1)} \in \mathbb{R}^{I_1 \times I_{23}}, \ \mathcal{X}_{(2)} \in \mathbb{R}^{I_2 \times I_{13}}, \ \mathcal{X}_{(3)} \in \mathbb{R}^{I_3 \times I_{12}} \tag{6}$$

for $I_{12} = I_1 \cdot I_2$, $I_{23} = I. I_3$ and $I_{13} = I_1 \cdot I_3$, where the column vectors of $\mathcal{X}_{(j)}$ are the j-mode vectors of $\mathcal{X}$ for $i = 1, 2, 3$. We express the j-mode unfolding

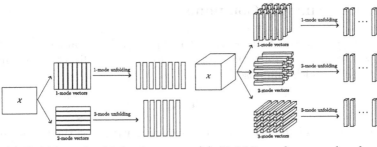

(a) Unfolding of a third order tensor

(b) Unfolding of a second order tensor

Fig. 3. Unfolding of tensors. (a) Unfolding for a second-order tensor. For a tensor in $\mathbb{R}^{6\times 8}$, unfolding for 1- and 2-modes yields eight 1-mode vectors and six 2-mode vectors, respectively. (b) Unfolding for a third-order tensor. For a tensor in $\mathbb{R}^{4\times 5\times 3}$, unfoldings for 1-, 2- and 3-modes yields fifteen 1-mode vectors, twelve 2-mode vectors and twenty 3-mode vectors, respectively.

of $\mathcal{X}_i$ as $\mathcal{X}_{i,(j)}$. Figures 3(a) and (b) show unfolding procedures for second- and third-order tensors, respectively.

For matrices $\boldsymbol{U} = ((u_{ii'})) \in \mathbb{R}^{I_1\times I_1}$, $\boldsymbol{V} = ((v_{jj'})) \in \mathbb{R}^{I_2\times I_2}$ and $\boldsymbol{W} = ((w_{kk'})) \in \mathbb{R}^{I_3\times I_3}$, the n-mode products for $n = 1, 2, 3$ of a tensor $\mathcal{X}$ are the tensors with entries

$$x_{[1]ijk} = \sum_{i'=1}^{I_1} x_{i'jk}u_{i'i}, \ \ x_{[2]ijk} = \sum_{j'=1}^{I_2} x_{ij'k}v_{j'j}, \ \ x_{[3]ijk} = \sum_{k'=1}^{I_3} x_{ijk'}w_{k'k}, \quad (7)$$

where $(\mathcal{X})_{ijk} = x_{ijk}$ is the ijkth element of the tensor $\mathcal{X}$. The inner product of two tensors $\mathcal{X}$ and $\mathcal{Y}$ in $\mathbb{R}^{I_1\times I_2\times I_3}$ is

$$\langle \mathcal{X}, \mathcal{Y} \rangle = \sum_{i=1}^{I_1}\sum_{j=1}^{I_2}\sum_{k=1}^{I_3} x_{ijk}y_{ijk}. \quad (8)$$

Using this inner product, we have the Frobenius norm of a tensor $\mathcal{X}$ as $|\mathcal{X}|_F = \sqrt{\langle \mathcal{X}, \mathcal{X}\rangle}$. The Frobenius norm $|\mathcal{X}|_F$ of the tensor $\mathcal{X}$ satisfies the relation $|\mathcal{X}|_F = |f|_2$, where $|f|_2$ is the Euclidean norm of the vector $\boldsymbol{f}$.

Tensor Projections. To project a tensor $\mathcal{X}$ in $\mathbb{R}^{I_1\times I_2\times I_3}$ to the tensor $\mathcal{Y}$ in a lower-dimensional tensor space $\mathbb{R}^{P_1\times P_2\times P_3}$, where $P_n \leq I_n$, three projection matrices $\{\boldsymbol{U}^{(n)}\}_{n=1}^3$ for $\boldsymbol{U}^{(n)} \in \mathbb{R}^{I_n\times P_n}$ are required for $n = 1, 2, 3$. Using these three projection matrices, we have the tensor orthogonal projection such that

$$\mathcal{Y} = \mathcal{X} \times_1 \boldsymbol{U}^{(1)\top} \times_2 \boldsymbol{U}^{(2)\top} \times_3 \boldsymbol{U}^{(3)\top}. \quad (9)$$

This projection is established in three steps, where in each step, each n-mode vector is projected to a P_n-dimensional space by $\boldsymbol{U}^{(n)}$ for $n = 1, 2, 3$.

3   Tensor Principal Components

Setting the data matrix X to be $X = \begin{pmatrix} f_1 & f_2 & \cdots & f_m \end{pmatrix}$ for data vectors $\{f_i\}_{i=1}^m$ in $\mathbb{R}^N$, whose mean is zero, the K-L transform is established by computing $\hat{f}_i = U f_i$ for U which minimises

$$J_1 = |UX|_F^2 \tag{10}$$

with the condition $U^\top U = I_N$. The orthogonal matrix U is the minimiser of

$$J_{11} = |UX|_F^2 + (U^\top U - I)\Lambda, \tag{11}$$

where $\Lambda = Diag(\lambda_1, \lambda_2, \cdots, \lambda_N)$ for $\lambda_1 \geq \lambda_2 \geq \lambda_2 \geq \cdots \geq \lambda_N \geq 0$. The minimiser of Eq. (11) is the solution of the eigenmatrix problem

$$MU = U\Lambda, \quad M = XX^\top. \tag{12}$$

The row vectors of U are the principal components.

The compression of f_i to a low-dimensional linear subspace is achieved by computing the transform $P_n U f$, where P_n is the orthogonal projection such that

$$P_n = \begin{pmatrix} I_n & O \\ O^\top & O \end{pmatrix} \tag{13}$$

for $n < N$.

For a collection of matrices $\{F_i\}_{i=1}^N \in \mathbb{R}^{m \times n}$ satisfying $E_i(F_i) = 0$, the orthogonal-projection-based data reduction $\hat{F}_i = U^\top F_i V$ is performed by maximising

$$J_2(U, V) = E_i \left(|U\hat{F}_i V^\top|_F^2 \right) \tag{14}$$

with respect to the conditions $U^\top U = I_m$ and $V^\top V = I_n$. The solutions are the minimiser of the Euler-Lagrange equation

$$J_{22}(U, V) = E \left(|U\hat{F}_i V^\top|_F^2 \right) + (I_m - U^\top U)\Sigma + (I_n - V^\top V)\Lambda. \tag{15}$$

Setting

$$\frac{1}{N} \sum_{i=1}^N F_i^\top F_i = M, \quad \frac{1}{N} \sum_{i=1}^N F_i F_i^\top = N, \tag{16}$$

U and V are the solutions of the eigendecomposition problems

$$MV = V\Lambda, \quad NU = U\Sigma, \tag{17}$$

where $\Sigma \in \mathbb{R}^{m \times m}$ and $\Lambda \in \mathbb{R}^{n \times n}$ are diagonal matrices satisfying the relationships $\lambda_i = \sigma_i$ for

$$\Sigma = \text{diag}(\sigma_1, \sigma_2, \ldots, \sigma_K, 0, \ldots, 0), \tag{18}$$
$$\Lambda = \text{diag}(\lambda_1, \lambda_2, \ldots, \lambda_K, 0, \ldots, 0). \tag{19}$$

The equation

$$(P_1 U)^\top X (P_2 V) = Y \tag{20}$$

is rewritten as

$$(P_2 V \otimes P_1 U)\mathrm{vec}X$$
$$= (P_2 \otimes P_1)(V \otimes U)X = P\mathrm{vec}X = \mathrm{vec}Y. \tag{21}$$

Using three projection matrices $U^{(i)}$ for $i = 1, 2, 3$, we have the tensor orthogonal projection for a third-order tensor as

$$\mathcal{Y} = \mathcal{X} \times_1 U^{(1)\top} \times_2 U^{(2)\top} \times_3 U^{(3)\top}. \tag{22}$$

For a collection $\{\mathcal{X}_k\}_{k=1}^m$ of the third-order tensors, the orthogonal-projection-based dimension reduction procedure is achieved by maximising the criterion

$$J_3 = E_k(|\mathcal{X}_k \times_1 U^{(1)} \times_2 U^{(2)} \times_3 U^{(3)}|_F^2) \tag{23}$$

with respect to the conditions $U^{(i)^\top} U^{(i)} = I$ for $i = 1, 2, 3$. The Euler-Lagrange equation of this conditional optimisation problem is

$$J_{33}(U^{(1)}, U^{(2)}, U^{(3)}) = E_k(|\mathcal{X}_k \times_1 U^{(1)} \times_2 U^{(2)} \times_3 U^{(3)}|_F^2)$$
$$+ \sum_{i=1}^3 |(I - U^{(i)^\top} U^{(i)})\Lambda^{(i)}|_F^2. \tag{24}$$

This minimisation problem is solved by the following iteration procedure.

1: $U_0^{(i)} := Q^{(i)}$ such that $Q^{(i)\top} Q^{(i)} = I$ and $\alpha = 0$.
2: $U_{(\alpha+1)}^{(1)} = arg \min J_{33}(U^{(1)}, U_{(\alpha)}^{(2)}, U_{(\alpha)}^{(3)})$.
3: $U_{(\alpha+1)}^{(2)} = arg \min J_{33}(U_{(\alpha+1)}^{(1)}, U^{(2)}, U_{(\alpha)}^{(3)})$.
4: $U_{(\alpha+1)}^{(3)} = arg \min J_{33}(U_{(\alpha+1)}^{(1)}, U_{(\alpha+1)}^{(2)}, U^{(3)})$.
5: if $|U_{(\alpha+1)}^{(i)} - U_{(\alpha)^i}|_F \leq \varepsilon$, then stop, else $\alpha := \alpha + 1$ and go to step 2.

For

$$J_{33}(U^{(1)}, U^{(2)}, U^{(3)}) = E_k(|\mathcal{X}_k \times_1 U^{(1)} \times_2 U^{(2)} \times_3 U^{(3)}|_F^2)$$
$$+ \sum_{i=1}^3 |(I - U^{(i)^\top} U^{(i)})\Lambda^{(i)}|_F^2, \tag{25}$$

setting $I := U_1^{(i)}$, the system of minimisation problems

$$U^{(1)} = arg \min f(U^{(1)}, I, I)$$
$$U^{(2)} = arg \min f(I, U^{(2)}, I) \tag{26}$$
$$U^{(3)} = arg \min f(I, I, U^{(3)})$$

is derived. This system of minimisation problem derives the following system of eigenmatrix probems,

$$
\begin{aligned}
\nabla_{U^{(1)}} J_{33}(U^{(1)}, I, I) &= 0 \\
\nabla_{U^{(2)}} J_{33}(I, U^{(2)}, I) &= 0 \\
\nabla_{U^{(3)}} J_{33}(I, I, U^{(3)}) &= 0.
\end{aligned}
\tag{27}
$$

From Eq. (27), as an extension of the two-dimensional problem, we define the system of optimisation problems

$$
J_j = E(|U^{(j)\top} \mathcal{X}_{i,(j)} U^{(j)}|_F^2) + (U^{(j)\top} U^{(j)} - I_j) \Lambda^{(j)}
\tag{28}
$$

for $i = 1, 2, 3$, as a relaxation of the iteration procedure, where $\mathcal{X}_{i,(j)}$ is the ith column vector of the unfolding matrix $\mathcal{X}_{(j)}$. These optimisation problems derive the system of eigenmatrix problems

$$
M^{(j)} U^{(j)} = U^{(j)} \Lambda^{(j)}, \quad M^{(j)} = \frac{1}{N} \sum_{i=1}^{N} \mathcal{X}_{i,(j)} \mathcal{X}_{i,(j)}^{\top}
\tag{29}
$$

for $j = 1, 2, 3$.

Setting $P^{(j)}$ to be an orthogonal projection in the linear space $\mathcal{L}(\{u_i^{(j)}\}_{i=1}^{I_j})$ spanned by the column vectors of $U^{(j)}$, data reduction is computed by

$$
\mathcal{Y} = \mathcal{X} \times_1 P^{(1)} U^{(1)} \times_2 P^{(2)} U^{(2)} \times_3 P^{(3)} U^{(3)}.
\tag{30}
$$

This expression is equivalent to the vector form

$$
vec\mathcal{Y} = (P^{(3)} \otimes P^{(2)} \otimes P^{(1)})(U^{(3)} \otimes U^{(2)} \otimes U^{(1)}) vec\mathcal{X}.
\tag{31}
$$

Dimensions of Subspaces. The eigenvalues of the eigenmatrices of Tucker-3 orthogonal decomposition satisfy the following theorem.

Theorem 1. *The eigenvalues of $U = U^{(1)} \otimes U^{(2)} \otimes U^{(3)}$ define a semi-order.*

Proof. For the eigenvalues $\lambda_i^{(1)}, \lambda_j^{(2)}, \lambda_k^{(3)}$ of the 1-, 2- and 3-modes of tensors, the inequalities $\lambda_i^{(1)} \lambda_j^{(2)} \lambda_k^{(3)} \geq \lambda_i^{(1)} \lambda_j^{(2)} \lambda_{k+1}^{(3)}$, $\lambda_i^{(1)} \lambda_j^{(2)} \lambda_k^{(3)} \geq \lambda_i^{(1)} \lambda_{j+1}^{(2)} \lambda_k^{(3)}$, $\lambda_i^{(1)} \lambda_j^{(2)} \lambda_k^{(3)} \geq \lambda_{i+1}^{(1)} \lambda_j^{(2)} \lambda_k^{(3)}$ define semi-orders among the eigenvalues. as

$$
\lambda_i^{(1)} \lambda_j^{(2)} \lambda_k^{(3)} \succeq \left\langle \lambda_i^{(1)} \lambda_j^{(2)} \lambda_{k+1}^{(3)}, \lambda_i^{(1)} \lambda_{j+1}^{(2)} \lambda_k^{(3)}, \lambda_{i+1}^{(1)} \lambda_j^{(2)} \lambda_k^{(3)} \right\rangle
\tag{32}
$$

is satisfied.   □

Regarding the selection of the dimension of the tensor subspace, Theorem 1 implies the following theorem.

Theorem 2. *The dimension of the subspace of the tensor space for data compression is $\frac{1}{6}n(n+1)(n+2)$ if we select n principal components in each mode of three-way array data.*

Proof. For a positive integer n, the number s_n of eigenvalues $\lambda_i^{(1)}\lambda_j^{(2)}\lambda_k^{(3)}$ is

$$s_n = \sum_{i+j+k=0,i,j,k\geq0}^{n-1} (i+j+k) = \sum_{l=1}^{n}\sum_{m=1}^{l} m = \frac{1}{6}n(n+1)(n+2).$$

$\square$

If $n = 1, 2, 3, 4$, we have $N = 1, 4, 10, 20$, respectively, for tensors $\mathcal{X} = ((x_{ijk}))$ in $\mathbb{R}^{I\times I\times I}$.

Setting $\{\boldsymbol{P}^{(i)}\}_{i=1}^3$ to be orthogonal projection matrices, the orthogonal projection of a third-order tensor $\mathcal{X}$ to the linear subspace Π_{123} by $\{\boldsymbol{P}^{(i)}\}_{i=1}^3$ is computed as

$$\mathcal{Y} = \mathcal{X} \times_1 \boldsymbol{P}^{(1)} \times_2 \boldsymbol{P}^{(2)} \times_3 \boldsymbol{P}^{(3)}. \tag{33}$$

Since $|\mathcal{Y}|_F$ is the length of the part of the tensor $\mathcal{X}$ on the linear subspace Π_{123}, the ratio $0 \leq |\mathcal{Y}|_F/|\mathcal{X}|_F \leq 1$ is the CCR of $\mathcal{X}$ to Π_{123}. The dimension of Π_{123} is computed by Theorems 1 and 2.

Graphical Truncation. For an approximated tensor $\hat{\mathcal{X}}_i$ of $\mathcal{X}_i$, we define the trancation operation

$$\hat{\mathcal{X}}_{i\Omega_i} = \begin{cases} \mathcal{O} \text{ if elements of } \mathcal{X} \text{ are zero} \\ \hat{\mathcal{X}} \text{ otherwise,} \end{cases} \tag{34}$$

to eliminate artefacts which appear in the background. For the graphical expression of $\hat{\mathcal{X}}_i$.

Discrete Cosine Transform and PCA. Since the discrete cosine transform (DCT) [16] is asymptotically equivalent to the matrix of the K-L transform [15] for data observed from a first-order Markov model [14,15], the dimension reduction by PCA is performed using the DCT as

$$f_{ijk}^n = \sum_{i'j'k'=0}^{n-1} g_{i'j'k'}\varphi_{i'i}\varphi_{j'j}\varphi_{k'k}, \; g_{ijk} = \sum_{i'j'k'=0}^{N-1} f_{i'j'k'}\varphi_{ii'}\varphi_{jj'}\varphi_{kk'} \tag{35}$$

for $n \leq N$, where

$$\boldsymbol{\Phi}_{(N)} = ((\epsilon\cos\frac{(2j+1)i}{2\pi N})) = ((\varphi_{ij})), \; \epsilon = \begin{cases} 1 & \text{if } j = 0 \\ \frac{1}{\sqrt{2}} & \text{otherwise} \end{cases} \tag{36}$$

is the DCT-II matrix of order N. If we apply the fast cosine transform to the computation of the 3D-DCT-II matrix, the computational complexity is $O(3N\log N)$.

In the vector and tensor forms, the transforms are expressed as

$$vec\mathcal{F}^n = (\boldsymbol{P}_{(3)} \otimes \boldsymbol{P}_{(2)} \otimes \boldsymbol{P}_{(1)})(\boldsymbol{\Phi}_{(N)} \otimes \boldsymbol{\Phi}_{(N)} \otimes \boldsymbol{\Phi}_{(N)})vec\mathcal{F} \qquad (37)$$

$$\mathcal{F}^n = \mathcal{F} \times_1 (\boldsymbol{P}_n^{(1)}\boldsymbol{\Phi}_{(N)}) \times_2 (\boldsymbol{P}_n^{(2)}\boldsymbol{\Phi}_{(N)}) \times_3 (\boldsymbol{P}_n^{(3)}\boldsymbol{\Phi}_{(N)}). \qquad (38)$$

Since $vec(\boldsymbol{u} \circ \boldsymbol{v} \circ \boldsymbol{w}) = \boldsymbol{u} \otimes \boldsymbol{v} \otimes \boldsymbol{w}$ the outer products of vectors redescribes the DCT-based transform as

$$\mathcal{F} = \sum_{i,j,k=1}^{N} a_{ijk}\boldsymbol{\varphi}_i \circ \boldsymbol{\varphi}_j \circ \boldsymbol{\varphi}_k, \; a_{ijk} = \langle \mathcal{F}, (\boldsymbol{\varphi}_i \circ \boldsymbol{\varphi}_j \circ \boldsymbol{\varphi}_k) \rangle \qquad (39)$$

where

$$\boldsymbol{\Phi}_{(N)} = (\boldsymbol{\varphi}_1, \boldsymbol{\varphi}_2, \cdots, \boldsymbol{\varphi}_N). \qquad (40)$$

The pyramid transform yields reduced images using the transform

$$g_{mn} = \sum_{i,j=-1}^{1} w_i w_j f_{2m-i\ 2n-j}, \qquad (41)$$

for $w_{\pm 1} = \frac{1}{4}$ and $w_0 = \frac{1}{2}$. This reduction g_{mn} from f_{mn} can be used as an outline of planar shapes.

Setting

$$\boldsymbol{R} = \frac{1}{2}(\boldsymbol{I} \otimes (0,1)^\top)(\boldsymbol{D} + 4\boldsymbol{I}) \qquad (42)$$

for the second order differential matrix $\boldsymbol{D}$, with the Neumann condition, such that,

$$\boldsymbol{D} = \begin{pmatrix} -1 & 1 & 0 & 0 & \cdots & 0 & 0 \\ 1 & -2 & 1 & 0 & \cdots & 0 & 0 \\ 0 & 1 & -2 & 1 & \cdots & 0 & 0 \\ \vdots & \vdots & \vdots & \vdots & \ddots & \vdots & \vdots \\ 0 & 0 & 0 & \cdots & 0 & 1 & -1 \end{pmatrix}, \qquad (43)$$

Eq. (41) is described as $\boldsymbol{G} = \boldsymbol{R}\boldsymbol{F}\boldsymbol{R}^\top$ for the image matrices $\boldsymbol{G}$ and $\boldsymbol{F}$.

Since the eigenmatrix of $\boldsymbol{D}$ is the DCT-II matrix, we have the following property.

Property 1. Setting $L^N =\mathsf{L}(\{\boldsymbol{\varphi}_k\}_{k=0}^{2^N-1})$, for two-dimensional images, the pyramid transform is a linear transform from $L^N \otimes L^N$ to $L^{\frac{N}{2}} \otimes L^{\frac{N}{2}}$.

Therefore, the dominant operation in the pyramid transform is the relaxed KL-transform using the DCT.

The three-dimensional pyramid transform

$$g_{pqr} = \sum_{i,j=-1}^{1} w_i w_j w_k f_{2p-i\ 2q-j\ 2r-k,,} \qquad (44)$$

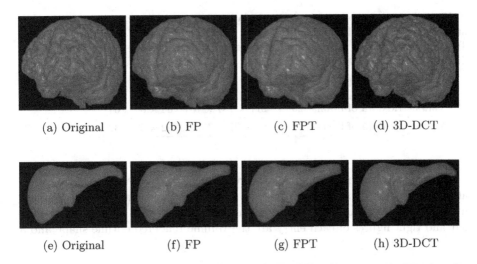

(a) Original   (b) FP   (c) FPT   (d) 3D-DCT

(e) Original   (f) FP   (g) FPT   (h) 3D-DCT

Fig. 4. Original and reconstructed volumetric data. From left to right, the first, second, third and fourth rows illustrate the original voxel images and results by the FP, FPT and 3D-DCT, respectively. (a)–(d) show volume renderings of voxel images of brains. (e)–(h) show volume renderings of voxel images of livers.

is re-described

$$\mathcal{Y} = \mathcal{X} \times_1 \boldsymbol{R} \times_2 \boldsymbol{R} \times_3 \boldsymbol{R} \tag{45}$$

using Tucker3 decomposition of $\mathcal{X}$. Moreover, the three-dimensional pyramid transform processes the following property.

Property 2. Setting $L^N = \mathsf{L}(\{\varphi_k\}_{k=0}^{2^N-1})$, for 3-dimensional images, the pyramid transform is a linear transform from $L^N \otimes L^N \otimes L^N$ to $L^{\frac{N}{2}} \otimes L^{\frac{N}{2}} \otimes L^{\frac{N}{2}}$.

Equation (45) directly derives an outline shape of a volumetric shape by enforcing and inhibiting low- and high frequency parts, respectively, on the DCT of the volumetric shape.

4   Numerical Examples

Setting the number of bases to be the size of the original tensors, we call the method the full projection (FP). If the number of selected bases is smaller than the size of the original tensors, we call the method the full projection truncation (FPT). For data compression using the FP, FPT and 3D-DCT, we adopt 20 volumetric simulation-brains generated by MRI simulation by BrainWeb [17] and liver data designed in Computational Anatomy project [18].

Table 1 shows the original size of the volumetric data and the reduced data size. The compression based on the FP, FPT and 3D-DCT the reduced sizes of a brain and liver $32 \times 32 \times 32$ and $64 \times 64 \times 64$ voxels, respectively.

Table 1. Sizes and numbers of volumetric data of brains and livers. ♯data represents the numbers of livers and brains. The data size is the original size of the volumetric data. The reduced data size is the size of the volume data after tensor-representation-based dimension reduction.

	♯data	Data size [voxel]	Reduced data size [voxel]
Volumetric data of brains	20	$217 \times 181 \times 181$	$64 \times 64 \times 64$
Volumetric data of livers	32	$89 \times 97 \times 76$	$32 \times 32 \times 32$

Figure 4 illustrates volumetric data reconstructed from reduced data generated by these three methods. Figures 5 and 6 illustrates the compressed volumetric data and their slices for brain and liver respectively. In each figure, the left and right figures of each entry are the volume-rendered outline shape and a

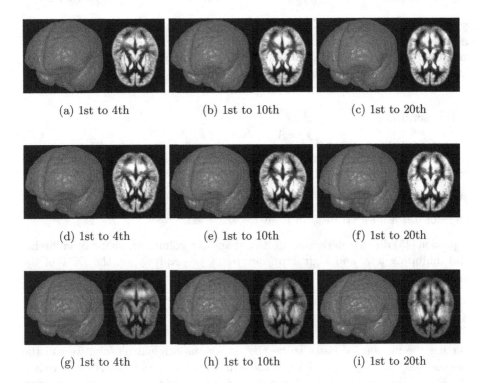

(a) 1st to 4th   (b) 1st to 10th   (c) 1st to 20th

(d) 1st to 4th   (e) 1st to 10th   (f) 1st to 20th

(g) 1st to 4th   (h) 1st to 10th   (i) 1st to 20th

Fig. 5. Compressed volumetric brain data and their slices. For the compressed volumetric brain data, we applied TPCA. For compression, we adopted the FP, FPT and 3D-DCT. The left and right figures of each entry are the volume-rendered outline shape and a slice of the volumetric data, respectively. From top to bottom, the results computed by the FP, FPT and 3D-DCT are illustrated. From left to right, results reconstructed using the 4, 10 and 20 principal major components of the TPCA are shown. The 80th axial slice of volumetric data is shown for each result.

slice of volumetric data, respectively. From top to bottom, the results computed by the FP, FPT and 3D-DCT are illustrated. From left to right, results using the 4, 10 and 20 principal major components of TPCA are shown. The 80th axial slice of volumetric data is shown for each result.

Figure 7 shows the CCR of the reordered eigenvalues of the FP for the projected tensors. As shown in Fig. 7, among the three methods, the CCRs from the first to the 20th eigenvalues are almost the same. In Fig. 5, the outline shapes of the reconstructed volumetric data are almost the same for the three methods.

These results indicate that the outline-shape extraction by the 3D-DCT is a relaxation of the TPCA. Moreover, the comparisons among results in Fig. 4 suggests that the principal major components reconstruct the outline shape of the volumetric data and the principal minor components reconstruct the interior texture of volume data.

Our numerical results show that, for a pair of small positive constants ε and δ, the relations

$$P(|\mathcal{Y}_\infty - \mathcal{Y}_\Phi|_F < \varepsilon) > 1 - \delta, \ P(|\mathcal{Y}_\infty - \mathcal{Y}|_F < \varepsilon)1 - \delta \qquad (46)$$

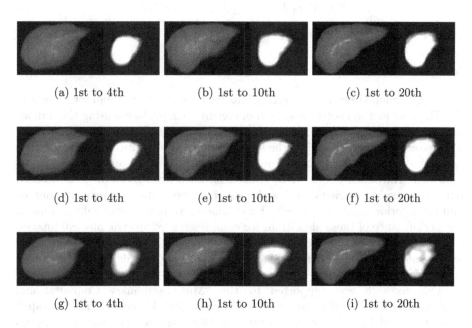

(a) 1st to 4th   (b) 1st to 10th   (c) 1st to 20th

(d) 1st to 4th   (e) 1st to 10th   (f) 1st to 20th

(g) 1st to 4th   (h) 1st to 10th   (i) 1st to 20th

Fig. 6. Compressed volumetric liver data and their slices. For the compressed volumetric data, we applied TPCA. For compression, we adopted the FP, FPT and 3D-DCT. The left and right figures of each entry are the volume-rendered outline shape and a slice of volumetric data, respectively. The results computed by FP are illustrated. From left to right, results reconstructed using the 4, 10 and 20 principal-major components of TPCA ares shown. The 80th axial slice of volumetric data is shown for each result.

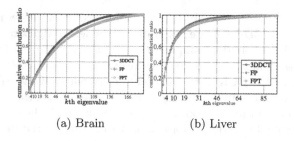

(a) Brain   (b) Liver

Fig. 7. CCR of TPCA for reduced volume data. For the compression, we adopted FP, FPT and 3D-DCT. For the computation of the CCR, we used all eigenvalues of modes 1, 2 and 3 after sorting the eigenvalues in decreasing order.

are satisfied based on the probabilistic correctness property for

$$\mathcal{Y}_\infty = \mathcal{X} \times_1 PU^{(1)}_{(\infty)} \times_2 PU^{(2)}_{(\infty)} \times_3 PU^{(3)}_{(\infty)} \tag{47}$$

$$\mathcal{Y}_\Phi = \mathcal{X} \times_1 P\Phi_{(N)} \times_2 P\Phi_{(N)} \times_3 P\Phi_{(N)} \tag{48}$$

$$\mathcal{Y} = \mathcal{X} \times_1 PU^{(1)} \times_2 PU^{(2)} \times_3 PU^{(3)}, \tag{49}$$

where $U^{(i)}_{(\infty)} = \lim_{\alpha \to \infty} U^{(i)}$ for $i = 1, 2, 3$.

5   Conclusions

We have developed two relaxed algorithms for tensor principal component analysis. The first method solves a system of eigenmatrix problems using the unfolding of a tensor, instead of solving a variational optimisation problem iteratively. The second method is based on the low-pass filtering of multidimensional signals using the discrete cosine transform (DCT), since the DCT efficiently approximates the Karhunen-Loève (K-L) transform. Such orthogonal-projection-based data compression extracts outline shapes of biomedical objects such as organs and the interior structures of cells. Furthermore, we have numerically evaluated the performance of these algorithms for compressing volumetric medical images.

The extension of the algorithms to higher order multi-way data analysis, such as the spatio-temporal volumetric analysis of moving and deforming objects is straightforward using higher-order tensors.

This research was supported by the "Multidisciplinary Computational Anatomy and Its Application to Highly Intelligent Diagnosis and Therapy" project funded by a Grant-in-Aid for Scientific Research on Innovative Areas from MEXT, Japan, and by Grants-in-Aid for Scientific Research funded by the Japan Society for the Promotion of Science.

References

1. Cichocki, A., Zdunek, R., Phan, A.-H., Amari, S.: Nonnegative Matrix and Tensor Factorizations: Applications to Exploratory Multi-way Data Analysis and Blind Source Separation. Wiley, Hoboken (2009)

2. Itskov, M.: Tensor Algebra and Tensor Analysis for Engineers. Springer, Heidelberg (2013)
3. Mørup, M.: Applications of tensor (multiway array) factorizations and decompositions in data mining. Wiley Interdisc. Rev.: Data Mining Knowl. Discov. **1**, 24–40 (2011)
4. Weber, G.W., Bookstein, F.L.: Virtual Anthropology: A Guide to a New Interdisciplinary Field. Springer, Heidelberg (2011)
5. Kroonenberg, P.M.: Applied Multiway Data Analysis. Wiley, Hoboken (2008)
6. Zelditch, M.L., Swiderski, D.L., Sheets, H.D.: Geometric Morphometrics for Biologists: A Primer, 2nd edn. Academic Press, Cambridge (2012)
7. Younes, L.: Shapes and Diffeomorphisms. Springer, Heidelberg (2010)
8. Davies, R., Twining, C., Taylor, C.: Statistical Models of Shape Optimisation and Evaluation. Springer, Heidelberg (2008)
9. Thompson, D.W.: On Growth and Form (The Complete Revised Edition). Dover, Minoela (1992)
10. Imiya, A., Eckhardt, U.: The Euler characteristics of discrete objects and discrete quasi-objects. CVIU **75**, 307–318 (1999)
11. Sakai, T., Narita, M., Komazaki, T., Nishiguchi, H., Imiya, A.: Image hierarchy in Gaussian scale space. In: Advances in Imaging and Electron Physics, vol. 165, pp. 175–263. Academic Press (2013)
12. Inagaki, S., Itoh, H., Imiya, A.: Multiple alignment of spatiotemporal deformable objects for the average-organ computation. In: Agapito, L., Bronstein, M.M., Rother, C. (eds.) ECCV 2014. LNCS, vol. 8928, pp. 353–366. Springer, Cham (2015). doi:10.1007/978-3-319-16220-1_25
13. Grenander, U., Miller, M.: Pattern Theory: From Representation to Inference. Oxford University Press, Oxford (2007)
14. Hamidi, M., Pearl, J.: Comparison of the cosine Fourier transform of Markov-1 signals. IEEE ASSP **24**, 428–429 (1976)
15. Oja, E.: Subspace Methods of Pattern Recognition. Research Studies Press, Baldock (1983)
16. Strang, G., Nguyen, T.: Wavelets and Filter Banks, 2nd edn. Wellesley-Cambridge Press, Wellesley (1996)
17. Aubert-Broche, B., Griffin, M., Pike, G.B., Evans, A.C., Collins, D.L.: 20 new digital brain phantoms for creation of validation image data bases. IEEE TMI **25**, 1410–1416 (2006)
18. http://www.comp-anatomy.org/wiki/index.php?Computational

Shape Preservation Based on Gaussian Radial Basis Function Interpolation on Human Corpus Callosum

Umut Orcun Turgut[✉] and Didem Gokcay

Informatics Institute, METU, Ankara, Turkey
umut.turgut@gmail.com, didemgokcay@gmail.com

Abstract. The Corpus Callosum (CC) has been a structure of much interest in neuroimaging studies of normal brain development, schizophrenia, autism, bipolar and unipolar disorder. In this paper, we present a technique which allows us to develop a shape preservation methodology in the deformation of CC for further global and regional shape analyzes between two sample corpora callosa. Source and target CC are superpositioned individually from eleven anchor points. Source CC is deformed in order to get superpositioned onto the target CC from these anchor points and superposition operation leads other anatomical landmarks to get placed automatically in all of the regions of source CC for further deformation analysis. Region construction via quadratic Bézier curves, deformation by using Gaussian RBF and quantifying the amount of deformation via generalized Procrustes analysis are used to infer the proper parameters used in minimum deformation. Amount of deformation can be analyzed both regionally and globally.

Keywords: Shape preserving interpolation · Radial Basis Functions · Space deformation

1 Introduction

Investigating the regional differences between samples of Corpus Callosum (CC) is a widely observed task in morphological studies. The gold standard in these kinds of studies is the works performed by the anatomists. For instance an anatomist may only describe the slightly thinned splenium between two corpora callosa in the right manner by just checking the MRI data. Currently there is no such an anatomic system which can point out this kind of anatomical difference into a semantic description like the one anatomist performs.

Shape is a property that keeps its characteristics when rotated or translated. Scaling and shearing make the shape of objects alter. In order to perform a prosperous regional comparison between two corpora callosa, a superposition operation that will align the source CC onto the target CC is needed to be carried out. The superposition operation should be performed from the handle points that are pointing anatomically to the same location in both structures.

© Springer International Publishing AG 2016
M. Reuter et al. (Eds.): SeSAMI 2016, LNCS 10126, pp. 118–132, 2016.
DOI: 10.1007/978-3-319-51237-2_10

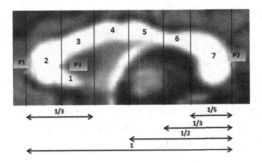

Fig. 1. Regional subdivision of the CC according to the study [15]. Parcellation landmarks are displayed as cyan circles. (Color figure online)

Those points are the key components of our mathematical model. For a near accurate comparison, shape deformation in this process must be minimal and the source structure should preserve its shape as much as possible after deformation.

In [15], author proposes an approach to define the regions of CC according to the anatomical connectivity. Figure 1 is showing the seven regional subdivisions, numbered 1 to 7, that will be also used in this study. P1 and P2 indicate the anteriormost and posteriormost points of the callosum with P1-P2 defined as the length of the callosum. Point P3 is the anteriormost point on the inner convexity of the anterior callosum. P1-P2 line is used as the linear axis to subdivide the callosum into anterior and posterior halves; anterior, middle, and posterior thirds; and the posterior one-fifth region (region 7). The line passing through P3, that is also perpendicular to the to the P1-P2 axis is used for defining the anteriormost division of the CC which generates regions rostrum (region 1) and genu (region 2). Region 3 is called as rostral body and it is the anteriormost one-third of the CC minus regions 1 and 2. Region 4 is called as anterior midbody and it is defined as the anterior one-half minus the anterior one-third. As for region 5, it is posterior midbody and is defined as the posterior one-half minus the posterior one-third. Region 6 is isthmus and it is defined as the posterior one-third minus the posterior one-fifth. Regions 3, 4, 5 and 6 constitute the body of the callosum. Regions, their anatomical labels and the callosal fibres in relation to cortical regions of origin and termination is displayed in Table 1.

The deformation function f basically maps the points p in the source CC to the new coordinates q; thus making the structure deformed. The deformation function needs to be built carefully and must hold the following properties [11]:

- Interpolation: The handle points p should map directly to q under deformation. (i.e. $f(p_i) = q_i$)
- Smoothness: f should produce smooth deformations
- Identity: If the deformed handles q are the same as p, then f should be the identity function. (i.e. $q_i = p_i \Rightarrow f(v) = v$)

These properties are similar to the ones that are used in the scattered data interpolation. In this paper, we introduce a deformation function that holds the all requirements covered above. Source CC is superpositioned onto the target CC from some handle points under the mathematical model of Gaussian Radial Basis Function (RBF). A mathematical model which maps the handle points of the source CC to anatomically the same handle points of target CC is calculated. Apart from these handle points, the model also affects the rest of the points on the boundary of source CC; thus making a deformation on the source CC shape. Our aim in this study is proposing a robust method for nearly preserving the characteristics of source CC shape after by localizing the deformations instead of globally deforming the whole CC.

Table 1. CC regions displayed in Fig. 1 and their anatomical locations [15].

Region	Anatomical label	Cortical region
1	Rostrum	Caudal/orbital prefrontal, inferior premotor
2	Genu	Prefrontal
3	Rostral body	Premotor, supplementary motor
4	Anterior midbody	Motor
5	Posterior midbody	Somaesthetic, posterior parietal
6	Isthmus	Superior temporal, posterior parietal
7	Splenium	Occipital, inferior temporal

Contributions. We offer a non-linear space deformation technique which lacks a cage that has to be defined before the interactive deformation operations start. Eleven handle points scattered through the borders of seven regions in CC replaces the cage and these handle points are defined semi-automatically via our framework. Our technique offers a simple formulation and is specific to the input shape which calculates the right parameters for minimal deformation and surface detail preservation for further comparison operations. In addition, it can be extended to 3D neuroanatomical structure studies with the proper anatomical anchor points. Our method is robust and efficient.

This paper is organized as follows: In the next section we address the related works; in Sect. 3, we describe the mathematical model; Sect. 4 includes the functionalities that can be included to the study and lastly in Sect. 5 future work is presented.

2   Related Work

Shape manipulation studies are performed under two categories, namely space deformation methods and surface-based methods. In the space deformation methods, the space that holds the object is deformed and hereby deforms the shape. As for the other one, shape deformation is carried out by using the object solely.

Space deformation techniques are much simpler and require less computational cost than surface-based methods since the deformation is carried out on the space that surrounds the mesh of the object rather than the mesh itself. They have less control on the shape detail preservation. Surface-based methods; however, depend on the mesh that wraps up the object; therefore, mesh quality becomes an important factor in these kinds of studies. The main advantage of the surface-based methods is the detail preservation on the shape. Due to this property, systems of surface-based methods are computationally expensive.

Zohar Levi et al. [6] offered a space deformation framework for real-time shape deformation which does not have a major effect on the local shape and volume. The technique for deformation is controlled locally and does not have an influence on the nearby branches. It is based on Interior Radial Basis Functions (IRBF) and local distortions are minimized by minimizing the distortion of a set of spheres that are placed within the object. Another space deformation technique that is based on triharmonic radial basis functions for real-time freeform shape editing is proposed in the study of Botsch et al. [2]. In this study, the desired target shape is not exactly defined before the deformation process starts. The deformation is put into practice in an interactive manner.

Using a predefined skeleton and free-form deformation (FFD) are also the popular space-deformation methods that have been used in shape manipulation studies. In the former one, the user defines a skeleton to the shape and the system adjusts the shape relative to the skeleton [7]. It has some disadvantages on the objects which structurally do not have any skeleton such as jellies. A sequence of lattices which converge to a region in 3D is created in an FFD study [10]. Each point is associated with a lattice. As the points in the lattice are modified, a deformation of the space is created, and the embedded points are relocated within that deformed space.

A space deformation method that is called as cage-based Variational Harmonic Map (VHM) is suggested by Ben-Chen et al. [1]. In this technique, manual editing of the cage is replaced by controlling it with intuitive positional and rotational constraints that are enforced through energy minimization, which optimizes the deformation rigidity and smoothness. Sederberg et al. proposed a method that includes a control lattice for shape deformation [12]. Lattices are proved to be problematic for controlling the articulated objects.

Mean Value Coordinates (MVC), Harmonic Coordinates (HC) and Green Coordinates (GC) are three forms of cage-based space deformation methods. A cage is a polyhedron which has a similar shape to the enclosed object. The points inside the cage are represented by affine sums of the cage's vertices multiplied by special weight functions. Manipulation on the cage makes its interior get deformed smoothly. The work presented in the study [8] is a cage-based technique which builds upon the positive MVC. These coordinates are used for mesh deformation. A similar study that is replacing the MVC with HC is proposed in the study [5]. This replacement makes each cage vertex non-negative and falls off with distance as measured within the cage. GCs that are derived from Green functions introduce appropriate rotations into the space deformation in order to allow shape preservation [9]. Weber et al. shows that GCs in the study [9] are a special case of complex barycentric coordinates and provides a simple analytic formula for them. Also an improvement on the GC is carried out and a new complex barycentric coordinates for 2D shape deformation is proposed in which the deformation better fits the user's specifications [14].

In the study of [13], the deformation is defined using a deformation graph which roughly conforms to the input shape. Deformation graphs are consisting of a varying number of nodes that the total size is related to the types of the edits that are going to take place. Coarse edits need fewer nodes than the detailed ones. An affine deformation is associated with each node in the deformation graph, which describes the transformation this node undergoes. The problem is stated as 'embedded deformation' since the algorithm must deform space through direct manipulation of objects within it, while preserving the embedded objects' features. Botsch et al. [3] puts forth a volumetric approach that is originated from the elastic energies of solid objects. The shape is break into voxels and the deformation is defined on them.

Igarishi et al. [4] proposes a point-based (surface-based) image deformation technique which results in a deformation that is called 'rigid-as-possible'. In this work, the amount of local scaling and shearing of deformations is minimized. The method is based on triangulation of the image and solving a linear system of equations whose size is equal to the number of vertices in the triangulation. In the study, the movement of vertices affects the positions of the other vertices in a way which results in a minimum distortion of each relevant triangle. Schaefer et al. [11] takes as a base of the study [4] and accelerates the deformations by solving a small linear system at each point in a uniform grid. This results in a very fast deformation of grids comprising tens of thousands of vertices in real time. Three classes of linear functions (affine, similarity and rigid) are used in the deformation method which is based on moving least squares.

Table 2. Points used in superposition operation and their anatomical locations.

Anchor point	Anatomical location
IP1	Intersection of regions rostrum & rostral body
IP2	Intersection of regions rostrum & genu
IP3	Intersection of regions genu & rostral body
IP4	Intersection of regions rostral body & anterior midbody (superior)
IP5	Intersection of regions anterior midbody & posterior midbody (superior)
IP6	Intersection of regions posterior midbody & isthmus (superior)
IP7	Intersection of regions isthmus & splenium (superior)
IP8	Intersection of regions isthmus & splenium (inferior)
IP9	Intersection of regions posterior midbody & isthmus (inferior)
IP10	Intersection of regions anterior midbody & posterior midbody (inferior)
IP11	Intersection of regions rostral body & anterior midbody (inferior)

The work presented here belongs to the space deformation category. Our main goal is to minimize the local deformations, thus to keep the localized characteristics of source CC regions, while superposing two corpora callosa for shape comparison. In this manner accurate semantic definition from the operation may be inferred. RBF is used for the deformation model where Gaussian is the basis function of the model. Eleven intersection points of seven callosal regions are defined as anchor points which are RBF centers at the same time. Anchor point decision affects the shape of deformation substantially. Decided points should be the same anatomical locations of corpora callosa for an efficient regional comparison. Apart from the number of total anchor points, the variance values of anchor points also affect the amount of deformation. Landmarks on the CC segments may be affected from just one anchor point or a combination of several anchor points. Proper variance values for each anchor point is one of the key studies of our work. These anchor points are summarized in Table 2 and displayed as orange circles in Fig. 2. Anchor points on the target CC are the final points that the initial ones will converge with the appropriate RBF weights. These weights are calculated according to the model. Proper weight value for each RBF center is decided after an iterative job which in the end lasts in a minimum localized source CC deformation. An error function is sum of squares of the difference between the actual source CC landmark coordinate before deformation and the one after deformation. The higher the function value, the more is the deformation. Therefore, error function searches for the proper weight values. General Procrustes Analysis (GPA) is used for calculating the morphological difference between two structures in this iterative job.

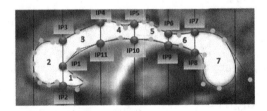

Fig. 2. Anchorage points for the superposition operation. (Color figure online)

Our method is basically as follows;

i. Source and target CC are parcellated into regions semi-automatically, in the guidance of the study [15].
ii. Manual shape modeling via quadratic Bézier curves is performed after regional parcellation.
iii. Source CC is superpositioned onto the target CC from the anchor points by the use of Gaussian RBF and a mathematical model is calculated.
iv. The parameters of the model are investigated with a method that is similar to Expectation Maximization (EM) for the minimum source CC deformation.

3   Shape Preservation with Gaussian RBF Interpolation

3.1   CC Parcellation

Samples of corpora callosa that are going to be investigated for regional differences are parcellated into compartments as an initial work. This process is performed semi-automatically in which three landmarks are needed to be manually defined on each CC image that has been loaded to the frame. The system then automatically divides the CC into seven regions as defined in the study [15]. Table 3 shows the points needed to parcellate the CC.

The boundaries of the callosal regions are calculated automatically with the positions of user defined landmarks and borders on the model are drawn. The whole operation lasts less than a minute for each CC. Figure 1 displays the segmented CC according to these parcellation landmarks. According to experimental work with monkeys and from postmortem studies of humans, a rough topography of callosal fibres in relation to cortical regions of origin and termination is displayed in Table 1.

3.2   CC Modeling

Quadratic Bézier curves are the building blocks of the modeling process. All of the callosal curves are represented with them.

A Bézier curve, specified by $n+1$ control points, is a parametric curve segment of order n. It is defined according to a parameter t over the interval $0 \leq t \leq 1$ and is formally expressed according to the polynomial series;

$$B(t) = \sum_{i=0}^{n} b_i B_{i,n}(t) \tag{1}$$

where $b0$, $b1$, . . . , bn are the control points of the curve and;

$$B_{i,n}(t) = \begin{cases} \frac{n!}{(n-i)!i!}(1-t)^{n-i}t^i & 0 \leq i \leq n \\ 0 & otherwise \end{cases} \tag{2}$$

are the Bernstein polynomials.

A curve segment is defined manually by defining these control points on the interface. User basically clicks on the frame and when the count of control point number reaches three, a quadratic Bézier curve is automatically formed according to the Eq. 1 and drawn on the interface. A region may consist of several Bézier curves and all of the curves are continuously connected to the adjacent curve segments. There is no gap either locally in a region or between the two adjacent callosal regions. Fine tuning of the user drawn segments is performed by just moving the control points of the Bézier curve segment. All seven regions are constructed in an anterior-posterior axis starting from the Rostrum.

Modeling operation lasts longer than parcellation. Each region needs seperate modeling. Thus, whole operation may last up to 7–8 minutes for each CC.

Table 3. Parcellation landmarks of the CC.

User defined points	Anatomical definition
P1	Anteriormost point of the CC
P2	Posteriormost point of the CC
P3	Inner convexity of the anterior CC

This may be the major drawback of our method if a large data set is under study. For a more powerful method, the modeling operation should be performed automatically.

Regional construction of callosal curves on the CC which is shown on Fig. 1 is displayed in Fig. 3.

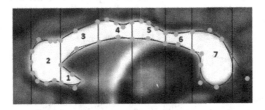

Fig. 3. Regional construction of callosal curves on the CC of Fig. 1. (Control polygons of each quadratic Bzier curve segment are displayed with blue dotted lines.) (Color figure online)

3.3   Regional Landmark Determination

Landmarks are determined in particular to the callosal regions. Total number of the landmarks is related with the total length of the curve segments in that region. The more the total length is the more the count of regional landmarks.

Separate curve which comprises of several quadratic Bézier curve segments is the key point in the determination of landmarks. Separate curves of a single region do not join; they are totally disjoint. The landmark determination and distribution is accomplished in particular to these separate curves. Since identical regions of two corpora callosa will have the same number of separate curves, one-to-one correspondence will be set between these curves and landmark operations are carried out particularly. This operation is performed for all of the separate curves of the region that is under study.

Figure 4 shows the landmark distribution in two callosal regions, namely rostrum and genu. There is one separate curve for each region and the length of this separate curve is used as a parameter in deciding the total number of landmarks. Figure 4 (a) shows callosal regions of Subject1 where red spots are indicating the positions of landmarks whereas (b) shows the callosal regions of Subject5. Here, in this example, it is seen that, 12 landmarks are calculated

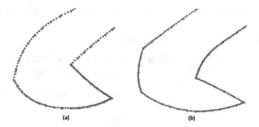

Fig. 4. Landmark distribution displayed in red on the segments of two callosal regions of **(a)** Subject1 **(b)** Subject5. (Color figure online)

for rostrum whereas 19 are for genu in both corpora callosa. There is one-to-one correspondence between these landmark pairs and all are used for further operations such as GPA.

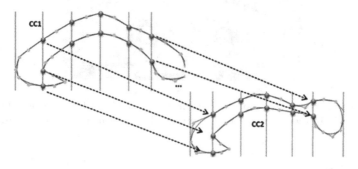

Fig. 5. One-to-one correspondence between the anchor points of two corpora callosa

3.4 Superposition

Superposition operation develops a mathematical model via the anchor points of source (CC1) and target (CC2) corpora callosa. This mathematical model is based on Gaussian RBF.

$$s(x) = a_0 + a_1 x + a_2 y + \sum_{i=1}^{N} \lambda i \phi(\|x - x_i\|) \tag{3}$$

where; $s(x)$ is the RBF, $\phi(r)$ is the basis function, $(r = \|x - x_i\|)$,$\|x\|$ is the Euclidean norm, the λ_i's are the RBF weights and the x_i's are the RBF centers.

The RBF consists of a weighted sum of a radially symmetric basic function $\phi(r)$ located at the centers x_i and a low degree polynomial $a_0 + a_1 x + a_2 y$. Given a set of N points x_i and values f_i, the process of finding an interpolating RBF is called fitting, such that:

$$s(x_i) = f_i, i = 1, 2, ..., N \tag{4}$$

The fitted RBF is defined by the λ_i, the coefficients of the basic function in the summation, together with the coefficients of the polynomial term $a_0 + a_1 x + a_2 y$.

RBF has proven to be an effective tool in multivariate interpolation problems of scattered data. Here in this operation, anchor points lying on the curve segments are the key components of the basis functions. There is a one-to-one correspondence from all of the eleven anchor points of CC1 to the CC2 as displayed in Fig. 5.

Weight Vector Calculation: Equation 4 can be rewritten in matrix form as a linear system;

$$Hw = b \tag{5}$$

$$H = \begin{bmatrix} \phi(||x_1 - x_1||) & \phi(||x_1 - x_2||) & \dots & \phi(||x_1 - x_N||) & 1 & x_1 & y_1 \\ \phi(||x_2 - x_1||) & \phi(||x_2 - x_2||) & \dots & \phi(||x_2 - x_N||) & 1 & x_2 & y_2 \\ \vdots & \vdots & \dots & \vdots & \vdots & \vdots & \vdots \\ 1 & 1 & \dots & 1 & 0 & 0 & 0 \\ x_1 & x_2 & \dots & x_N & 0 & 0 & 0 \\ y_1 & y_2 & \dots & y_N & 0 & 0 & 0 \end{bmatrix}$$

$$w^T = (\lambda_1, \lambda_2, \dots, \lambda_N, a_0, a_1, a_2)$$

$$b^T = (f_1, f_2, \dots, f_N, 0, 0, 0)$$

where the dimension of interpolation matrix H is $(N+3, N+3)$, weight matrix w is $(N+3, 1)$ and the result matrix b is $(N+3, 1)$. Solving the linear system (Eq. 5) determines λ_i's and a's. The RBF that is used in this study is Gaussian, that is;

$$\phi(r) = e^{(-(\frac{1}{2\sigma^2})r^2)} \tag{6}$$

where σ is the standard deviation value of the relevant RBF center. In our model RBF centers (x_i) are the eleven anchor points of CC1 (N is 11) whereas b's are the coordinates of anchor points of CC2. Interpolation matrix (H) is formed by taking into account of the eleven anchor points of CC1. Row values are calculated in particular to an anchor point. For example first row includes the Gaussian RBF function values of all eleven anchor points according to anchor point IP1. The last three columns in the same row are filled with the values of 1, x and y coordinate values of IP1, respectively. Likewise second row includes the Gaussian RBF values according to anchor point IP2, and so on. First eleven columns of the last three rows in the interpolation matrix includes values of 1, x and y coordinate values of IP$ where $ is equal to the column number. The 3×3 submatrix in the lower right corner is the zero matrix. When nonsingular H matrix is prepared, weight matrices which are going to be used in superposition operation are calculated according to the equations;

$$w_x = H^{-1}b_x, w_y = H^{-1}b_y \tag{7}$$

Deciding the New Coordinates: Weight matrices which are calculated in the previous step are used in calculating the new coordinates of every single point that forms the Bézier curve segments of CC1. Interpolation matrix H is prepared by the use of point which is going to be deformed on the CC1 and the eleven anchor points, as in Eq. 5. The dimension of the H matrix will be $(1, N + 3)$. While calculating the values of first eleven columns in the matrix H, standard deviation value of the relevant anchor point is used, as shown with $\sigma_{\$}$ symbol in Fig. 6.

(x, y) coordinate pair for all of the points on the Bézier curve segments of CC1 after deformation is calculated with the matrix multiplication of interpolation matrix H and w_x, interpolation matrix H and w_y, respectively.

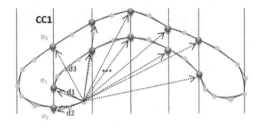

Fig. 6. Interpolation matrix (H) formation for calculating deformed coordinate pair.

Superposition Operation: The application of superposition operation requires basically determining anchor points and calculating mathematical model of the deformation.

The model that was prepared is applied to every points which form the regional curve segments. Carrying model into execution forms the deformed shape. Figure 7 shows **(a)** the source CC before deformation, **(b)** the target CC that the source is going to be superimposed on from the eleven anchor points, **(c)** the CC after deformation.

3.5   Minimum Deformation Calculation

The standard deviation value of each anchor points effects the outcome. Therefore, these values are treated as parameters to be learned. We run an iterative approach that is like the Expectation Maximization algorithm in mixture of Gaussians. This method makes us calculate different standard deviation values for each of the anchor points. As a result minimum deformation may be derived. Three step iterative approach is basically pointed out below.

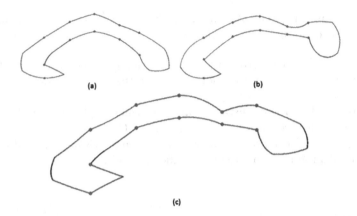

Fig. 7. Superposition operation. **(a)** CC before deformation **(b)** target CC to get anchored **(c)** CC after deformation via RBF model that is based on anchor points all of which have standard deviation values of 0.5 (red dots indicate the eleven anchor points). (Color figure online)

   i. Fix all standard deviation (σ) values and solve for weight vectors.
  ii. Fix weight vectors and minimize error function with respect to σ.
 iii. With newly calculated σ values, solve for weight vectors again.
 iv. Go to step i until maximum number of iterations is exceeded or difference of σ_i and σ_{i+1} are below a defined threshold value.

Our error function is the common sum-of-squares error, that is;

$$E(x) = \frac{1}{2}\sum_{k=1}^{c}(y_k(x) - t_k)^2 \tag{8}$$

The derivative of this error with respect to the standard deviation of basis function j, (σ_j), is;

$$\frac{\partial E}{\partial \sigma_j}(x) = \sum_k (y_k(x) - t_k) w_{kj} e^{\frac{\left\| (x-x_j)^2 \right\|}{2\sigma_j^2}} \frac{\left\| (x-x_j)^2 \right\|}{\sigma_j^3} \tag{9}$$

where c is the total number of landmarks on the CC boundary, $y_k(x)$ is the desired value and t_k is the actual value of that point.

$$\sigma_j = \sigma_j - n\frac{\partial E}{\partial \sigma_j} \tag{10}$$

where n is the learning rate.

4 Conclusion

37 source corpora callosa obtained from both normal subjects and subjects suffering from Major Depression Disorder (MDD) are studied according to the

model covered in this paper. Also an atlas CC is added as a target CC model to the study. The experiment is as follows;

i. Each source CC among 37 subjects is superimposed onto the target CC and proper parameters of all anchor points for the minimum deformation are obtained.
ii. 37 separate Procrustes distance value are calculated between the pairs of deformed source corpora callosa and target CC.
iii. The effect of deformation on the original source CCs is investigated via t-test whether it produces statistically significant results or not.

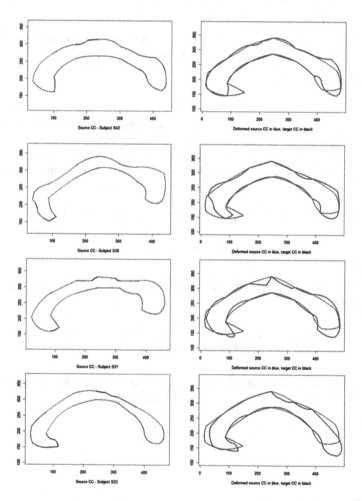

Fig. 8. Deformation operation. Source CC's are deformed according to the target CC via RBF that is holding proper parameters for each anchor points. (Color figure online)

Figure 8 shows sample deformations in our experiment. Each row belongs to a different subject and deformation is performed according to the same atlas. In the figure, CCs on the left show the original CCs of three subjects and CCs that are drawn with blue lines on the right show the deformed shapes of relevant CC. The black CCs on the right are the same target structure that is also called as atlas in the paper.

The null hypothesis (Ho) in our experiment basically assumes that deformation has no effect on the CC shapes whereas alternative hypothesis (Ha) claims that statistically significant difference occurs on the CC shape structures after deformation. Calculated t-value for the experiment becomes 15.86, which means Ho hypothesis is need to be rejected. As a conclusion, deformation changes the structures of source CCs significantly.

5   Discussion

Modeling the CC can be fully automated. This will outcome the automated parcellation; automated modeling of callosal regions which includes deciding on the number of segments that will form the callosal boundary, drawing Bézier curve segments and merging them.

Some preprocessing steps before the selection of anchor points may also be included into the study.

6   Future Work

The same experiment is going to be performed with the methods of affine Moving Least Squares (MLS), similarity MLS, rigid MLS, GC, MVC, HC and rigid-as-possible. The inner-distance values such as Floyd-Warshall or Johnson instead of Euclidean distance may also be applied in the relevant models and the results are going to be compared with the one that is obtained in our study.

References

1. Ben-Chen, M., Weber, O., Gotsman, C.: Variational harmonic maps for space deformation. ACM Trans. Graph. (TOG) **28**, 34 (2009)
2. Botsch, M., Kobbelt, L.: Real-time shape editing using radial basis functions. In: Computer Graphics Forum, vol. 24, pp. 611–621. Wiley Online Library (2005)
3. Botsch, M., Pauly, M., Wicke, M., Gross, M.: Adaptive space deformations based on rigid cells. In: Computer Graphics Forum, vol. 26, pp. 339–347. Wiley Online Library (2007)
4. Igarashi, T., Moscovich, T., Hughes, J.F.: As-rigid-as-possible shape manipulation. ACM Trans. Graph. (TOG) **24**, 1134–1141 (2005)
5. Joshi, P., Meyer, M., DeRose, T., Green, B., Sanocki, T.: Harmonic coordinates for character articulation. ACM Trans. Graph. (TOG) **26**, 71 (2007)
6. Levi, Z., Levin, D.: Shape deformation via interior RBF. IEEE Trans. Vis. Comput. Graph. **20**(7), 1062–1075 (2014)

7. Lewis, J.P., Cordner, M., Fong, N.: Pose space deformation: a unified approach to shape interpolation and skeleton-driven deformation. In: Proceedings of the 27th Annual Conference on Computer Graphics and Interactive Techniques, pp. 165–172. ACM Press/Addison-Wesley Publishing Co. (2000)
8. Lipman, Y., Kopf, J., Cohen-Or, D., Levin, D.: GPU-assisted positive mean value coordinates for mesh deformations. In: Symposium on Geometry Processing (2007)
9. Lipman, Y., Levin, D., Cohen-Or, D.: Green coordinates. ACM Trans. Graph. (TOG) **27**, 78 (2008)
10. MacCracken, R., Joy, K.I.: Free-form deformations with lattices of arbitrary topology. In: Proceedings of the 23rd Annual Conference on Computer Graphics and Interactive Techniques, pp. 181–188. ACM (1996)
11. Schaefer, S., McPhail, T., Warren, J.: Image deformation using moving least squares. ACM Trans. Graph. (TOG) **25**, 533–540 (2006)
12. Sederberg, T.W., Parry, S.R.: Free-form deformation of solid geometric models. ACM SIGGRAPH Comput. Graph. **20**(4), 151–160 (1986)
13. Sumner, R.W., Schmid, J., Pauly, M.: Embedded deformation for shape manipulation. ACM Trans. Graph. (TOG) **26**, 80 (2007)
14. Weber, O., Ben-Chen, M., Gotsman, C.: Complex barycentric coordinates with applications to planar shape deformation. In: Computer Graphics Forum, vol. 28, pp. 587–597. Wiley Online Library (2009)
15. Witelson, S.F.: Hand and sex differences in the isthmus and genu of the human corpus callosum. Brain **112**(3), 799–835 (1989)

Author Index

Printed in the United States
By Bookmasters